NUTRITION AND DIET RESEARCH PROGRESS

FRUCTOSE

SYNTHESIS, FUNCTIONS AND HEALTH IMPLICATIONS

NUTRITION AND DIET RESEARCH PROGRESS

Additional books in this series can be found on Nova's website under the Series tab.

Additional e-books in this series can be found on Nova's website under the e-books tab.

FOOD SCIENCE AND TECHNOLOGY

Additional books in this series can be found on Nova's website under the Series tab.

Additional e-books in this series can be found on Nova's website under the e-books tab.

NUTRITION AND DIET RESEARCH PROGRESS

FRUCTOSE

SYNTHESIS, FUNCTIONS AND HEALTH IMPLICATIONS

BRANDON M. JOHNSTON
AND
AARON B. COLLINS
EDITORS

Nova Science Publishers, Inc.
New York

For permission to use material from this book please contact us:
Telephone 631-231-7269; Fax 631-231-8175
Web Site: http://www.novapublishers.com

LIBRARY OF CONGRESS CATALOGING-IN-PUBLICATION DATA

ISBN: 978-1-62081-126-9
Library of Congress Control Number: 2012932535

Published by Nova Science Publishers, Inc. † New York

CONTENTS

Preface		**vii**
Chapter 1	Unhealthy Diet Intake during the Peri-Natal and Adult Periods: Detrimental Neuroendocrine and Metabolic Effects *Eduardo Spinedi, Andrés Giovambattista, Oscar R. Rebolledo, Rolf C. Gaillard and Juan J Gagliardino*	**1**
Chapter 2	High-Fructose Consumption and Metabolic Diseases *Cleide E. P. Trindade, Cilmery Kurokawa, Rodrigo C. Barreiros and Grasiela Bossolan*	**37**
Chapter 3	Fructose and Non-Alcoholic Fatty Liver Disease *Ting Zhang, Shen Qu, Steven Ringquist and H. Henry Dong*	**61**
Chapter 4	Detrimental Effects of Excessive Fructose Ingestion on Memory and Other Brain Functions *E. C. Bruggeman, A. P. Ross and M. B. Parent*	**81**
Chapter 5	Role of Fructose in Body Functions: An overview *N. Assy, F. Adawi and W. Nseir*	**101**
Chapter 6	Fructose Facilitates Alcohol Metabolism *I. Onyesom*	**117**
Chapter 7	Fructose and the Control of Food Intake *Danielle Colley, Edra London, Baijia Jiang, Jasjeet Khural and Thomas Castonguay*	**131**
Chapter 8	Effect Of Fructose On Health *Tzi Bun Ng, Jack Ho Wong, Evandro Fei Fang and Xiujuan Ye*	**145**
Chapter 9	Mammalian Triokinase and Dihydroxyacetone Kinase are the Same Enzyme *David J. Timson*	**153**
Index		**161**

PREFACE

Fructose is a carbohydrate found in plants and humans. It was isolated in 1947 from sugar cane, where it is a component of sucrose. In this book, the authors discuss the synthesis, functions and health implications of fructose. Topics include high-fructose consumption and metabolic disease; detrimental neuroendocrine and metabolic effects of fructose during peri-natal and adult periods; fructose and non-alcoholic fatty liver disease; and fructose ingestion effects on brain functions.

Chapter 1 - Consumption of unhealthy diets (so called "modern diets") in early/late life might play a key role in the development of obesity, metabolic syndrome (MS) and type 2 diabetes (T2DM). Due to the epidemic growth profile of these diseases with their negative socioeconomic impact, this unhealthy habit becomes a relevant preventive target factor to improve human longevity/life quality and to reduce the current economic load for the public health system worldwide. The authors have currently reviewed data from studies addressing the impact of the intake of an iso-caloric fructose-rich diet (FRD) by either lactating mothers or adult individuals on metabolic and endocrine adipose tissue (AT) functions. Data from several hypothalamic functions, peripheral metabolic markers, and the pattern of the AT adipokine production were also compiled from experiments performed in those two conditions. Since one of the most important derangements caused by the intake of an excess of fructose is an overall enhancement in oxidative stress (OS) rate, the studies revisited have explored both its indirect and direct consequences upon body weight, food intake, hypothalamic function, adipoinsular axis activity, and the sensitivity of various tissues to insulin and leptin stimuli. The role of the AT dysfunction generated after feeding individuals with a FRD has also been deeply examined. Data collected clearly indicate that the intake of a FRD triggers the development of several features similar to those found in the human phenotype of MS, e.g., hyperadiposity, impaired glucose tolerance, dyslipemia, insulin- and leptin-resistance, enhanced prothrombotic risk and dysfunction of the hypothalamic satiety signal. Moreover, the intake of this diet negatively affects several of the above mentioned functions regardless of whether this interventional diet is applied directly or indirectly and earlier or later to an organism over development. This evidence must help health policy makers to develop/implement appropriate strategies to promote healthy dietary habits in the general population to prevent the development of chronic diseases such as obesity and T2DM, thus improving the population life quality and decreasing the heavy load of these diseases upon health care budgets and society overall.

Chapter 2 - Renewed interest in the study of fructose arose after a number of papers on the harmful effects of ingesting high-fructose diets were published. Fructose intake has increased significantly in the United States and worldwide in the last four decades, which is mainly due to the increased consumption of high-fructose corn syrup and sucrose as a sweetener in beverages and in industrialized foods. There is substantial evidence from studies on rodents and on human adults suggesting that fructose intake in large amounts and for a long period of time leads to the development of the metabolic syndrome, insulin resistance, and dyslipidemia with increased plasma triacylglycerol, phospholipids and de novo lipogenesis. As a consequence, fructose may contribute to increased obesity, hypertension, type-2 diabetes and cardiovascular diseases. Fructose is a monosaccharide found in fruit, some vegetables and honey. Sucrose, a natural sweetener found in sugar cane and beets (50% fructose), is a disaccharide with two hexoses, one glucose molecule bonded to a fructose molecule by an alpha-1-4 glycoside. Although fructose has the same chemical formula as that of glucose ($C_6 H_{12} O_6$), it differs in its structure and metabolism. In the last few decades, sweeteners have been produced by corn starch hydrolysis, and part of the glucose produced is changed into fructose by enzymatic isomerization. This high-fructose corn syrup (42%-55% fructose) has a lower price than sucrose, and it has increasingly replaced sucrose as a sweetener in beverages and industrialized foods. Fructose can be produced from glucose by the sorbitol pathway. In endogenous fructose production, non-phosphorylated glucose is converted into fructose. Initially, glucose produces sorbitol in a reaction catalyzed by aldose reductase. In the next step, fructose is formed from sorbitol in a reaction catalyzed by sorbitol dehydrogenase. This pathway may be important in the embryonic stages of human life for regeneration of pyridine nucleotides in order to maintain ATP concentrations and cellular redox potentials when the fetus is in a low oxygen environment. After absorption, fructose is rapidly extracted by the liver and metabolized into fructose-1-phosphate in a reaction catalyzed by fructokinase, which is specific for fructose. Subsequently, fructose-1-P is split by fructose-1-phosphate aldolase in trioses, dihydroxyacetone phosphate and glyceraldehyde, a pathway to provide the backbone for triacylglycerol and phospholipid synthesis. Triose-P is converted into glucose and glycogen as well as into lactate, which can produce plasma lactic acidosis, and into glycerol, a precursor for triglycerides and de novo lipogenesis. Although considerable evidence suggests that high fructose intake can produce harmful effects, investigations where high-fructose diets are compared with high-glucose diets are necessary to clarify the real role played by free fructose in adverse metabolic effects. In epidemiological studies, the analysis of the effects of high-fructose corn syrup and high sucrose intake must consider that both products are composed of fructose and glucose.

Chapter 3 - Fructose is referred to as fruit sugar that is highly enriched in corn syrup. High fructose corn syrup is increasingly used as a sweetener in processed foods, baked goods, and carbonated soft drinks. High consumption of fructose is alleged as a causative factor for non-alcoholic fatty liver disease, a pathological condition that is characterized by excessive fat accumulation in the liver of individuals who drink little or no alcohol. It is puzzling as to how chronic consumption of refined fructose in carbonated beverages is associated with adverse effects, whereas daily intake of fructose-containing fruits and honey is considered beneficial for health. In this chapter, the authors will review the molecular mechanism by which fructose is metabolized in the body and provide unbiased view of whether fructose consumption is a risk factor for nonalcoholic fatty liver disease.

Chapter 4 - Fructose is a monosaccharide found naturally in fruits, honey, and some vegetables. It also is added to foods in the form of sucrose, concentrated fruit juices, corn syrup, high fructose corn syrup, and crystalline fructose. The addition of fructose to a wide variety of foods and beverages has led to a significant increase in fructose consumption over the past three decades. This is a cause for concern, because excessive intake of fructose causes a variety of pathological effects, including hypertriglyceridemia, visceral adiposity, hyperinsulinemia, non-alcoholic fatty liver disease (NAFLD), elevated inflammatory factors, insulin resistance, Type 2 diabetes, and hypertension/ cardiovascular disease. These physiological effects of a high fructose diet are well-documented; in contrast, relatively little is known about the effects of excessive fructose consumption on the central nervous system. The purpose of this chapter is to review the effects of high fructose intake in rodents on the brain, with a particular focus on plasticity and memory. Evidence implicating elevated triglyceride levels, NAFLD, neuroinflammation, and oxidative stress in the pathological effects of a high fructose diet on brain function is presented. Sex-dependent effects of elevated fructose consumption and application of results from experimental models of fructose consumption to the human population also are discussed.

Chapter 5 - The consumption of fructose has increased considerably in the world during the last decades. Excessive fructose consumption may be responsible in part for the increasing prevalence of obesity, non alcoholic fatty liver disease (NAFLD), metabolic syndrome, and diabetes mellitus. Fructose promotes the formation of toxic advanced glycation end-products (AGE'S), which appear to play a role in the development of atherosclerosis, aging process; and in the pathogenesis of vascular, renal and ocular complication of diabetes; Fructose has also been implicated as the main cause of symptoms in some patients with chronic diarrhea or other functional bowel disturbances (IBS). Although the long term effects of fructose consumption have not been adequately studied in humans, the available evidence suggests it may be more harmful than is generally recognized.

Chapter 6 - Alcohol is a clear, colourless, mobile, volatile, inflammable liquid with a characteristic spirituous, faint, sharp odour of burning taste formed by vinous fermentation. Chemically, alcohols are a group of organic compounds with hydroxyl (-OH) group attached to a hydrocarbon (R-) chain, generally represented as R-OH. The OH group determines the behaviour of alcohols. The alcohol contained in various alcoholic beverages (wine, beer, gin, whiskey, and spirits) is ethanol (C_2H_5OH), a small molecular weight, non-polar compound which does not require modification or digestion before absorption.

Chapter 7 - Over the past 3 years, the authors have generated several lines of evidence showing that fructose can exert influence over several physiological systems that are known to participate in the regulation of food intake. In particular, the authors have demonstrated that fructose consumption can rapidly influence intracellular glucocorticoid regulation in both liver and adipose tissue. Further, the authors have reported that fructose access leads to a modification of several genes in the hypothalamus that have been linked to appetite control. The basic experimental paradigm used for these observations was to give laboratory rats free access to food, water and one of several sugar solutions for 24 h or one week, after which blood and tissues were collected. The authors observed that overnight fructose access (as opposed to overnight access to other sugars) leads to an almost doubling of circulating triglycerides. Despite differences in the sugars and their respective metabolic consequences, 16% (w/v) solutions of glucose, fructose and sucrose were consumed in similar amounts. All groups given access to sugar consumed significantly more calories than did rats given chow only. Diets high in fructose, but not glucose or sucrose, increased 11β-HSD1 mRNA within 24 h in both liver and adipose by greater than two- and threefold, respectively ($P \leq 0.05$). Dopamine receptors 1a and 2 and neuropeptide Y (NPY) were upregulated in the hypothalami taken from the fructose fed rats when compared to rats fed only the control diet. Hypothalamic Galanin, Brs3, AGRP, INSR, Gh1, Trhr, Atrn, NMB, TNF and Thrb were downregulated in the fructose fed group compared to controls. Results of these experiments demonstrate that fructose can have very different effects on several of the mechanisms that control food intake and body weight when compared to the effects of glucose.

Chapter 8 - Fructose and fructose-based sweeteners are the most commonly added sugars in our diet. Fructose has both beneficial actions as well as harmful effects.Lactulose formed by lactose isomerization, stimulates the growth of health-promoting bacteria in the gastrointestinal tract, and suppresses proliferation of pathogenic bacteria. Calcium fructoborate reduces exacerbated cellular immune responses induced by mycotoxins from *Fusarium* species. Fructooligosaccharides have probiotic effect, improve mineral absorption, reduce constipation, and reduce serum levels of cholesterol, triacylglycerols and phospholipids. They are additives in some food products and infant formulas due to their probiotic effect. Fructose is a highly lipogenic nutrient implicated in insulin resistance, hepatic steatosis, and the metabolic syndrome. Fructose induces an increase in ethanol metabolism and elevates the risk of Syndrome X. A high-fructose diet aggravates eccentric left ventricular hypertrophy in experimental volume overload.The diet also results in development of hypertension. Excessive dietary carbohydrates, especially fructose, may promote the development of Alzheimer's disease. An excess of carbohydrates, such as fructose and chocolate, either during gestation or lactation, has an adverse effect on offspring.Maternal fructose intake during pregnancy and lactation alters placental growth and leads to sex-specific changes in fetal and neonatal endocrine function. The aqueous extract of *Globularia alypum* decreases hypertriglyceridemia and ameliorates oxidative status of the muscle, kidney, and heart in rats fed a high-fructose diet. Grape seed extract supplementation prevents high-fructose diet-induced insulin resistance in rats by improving insulin and adiponectin signalling pathways. Despite the evidence presented above, some investigators are of the opinion that there is insufficient evidence to support the prohibition or restriction of the use of high fructose corn syrup or other fructose-containing sweeteners or to advocate the use of warning labels on products containing high fructose corn syrup. Although some studies indicate that fructose does not bring about biologically relevant changes in triglyceride or body weight when consumed at levels near 95th percentile estimates of intake, it is advisable to restrict ingestion of caloric sweeteners, including high fructose corn syrup.

Chapter 9 - It is widely accepted that the ATP-dependent phosphorylation of D-glyceraldehyde in the fructokinase pathway of fructose metabolism requires the enzyme “triokinase”. However, experimental data on this enzyme are remarkably scarce. The enzyme has been purified from a variety of sources and peptides derived from the pig kidney enzyme show high similarity to human dihydroxyacetone kinase – an enzyme which also has FMN cyclase activity in high manganese ion concentrations. The properties of the two enzymes are also highly similar. Therefore it is proposed that mammalian triokinase and dihydroxyacetone kinase are, in fact, the same enzyme. This has consequences for investigations of normal and aberrant fructose metabolism and for the teaching of biochemistry in medical and science courses.

In: Fructose
Editors: Brandon M. Johnston and Aaron B. Collins
ISBN: 978-1-62081-126-9

Chapter 1

UNHEALTHY DIET INTAKE DURING THE PERI-NATAL AND ADULT PERIODS: DETRIMENTAL NEUROENDOCRINE AND METABOLIC EFFECTS

Eduardo Spinedi[1*], Andrés Giovambattista[1], Oscar R. Rebolledo[2], Rolf C. Gaillard [3+], and Juan J Gagliardino[2]

[1]Neuroendocrine Unit, Multidisciplinary Institute on Cell Biology (CONICET-CICPBA), La Plata, Argentina
[2]CENEXA, PAHO/WHO Collaborating Center for Diabetes (CONICET-UNLP), 1900 La Plata, Argentina and, [3]Division of Endocrinology, Diabetology and Metabolism, University Hospital, CH, Lausanne, Switzerland

ABSTRACT

Consumption of unhealthy diets (so called "modern diets") in early/late life might play a key role in the development of obesity, metabolic syndrome (MS) and type 2 diabetes (T2DM). Due to the epidemic growth profile of these diseases with their negative socioeconomic impact, this unhealthy habit becomes a relevant preventive target factor to improve human longevity/life quality and to reduce the current economic load for the public health system worldwide. We have currently reviewed data from studies addressing the impact of the intake of an iso-caloric fructose-rich diet (FRD) by either lactating mothers or adult individuals on metabolic and endocrine adipose tissue (AT) functions. Data from several hypothalamic functions, peripheral metabolic markers, and the pattern of the AT adipokine production were also compiled from experiments performed in those two conditions. Since one of the most important derangements caused by the intake of an excess of fructose is an overall enhancement in oxidative stress (OS) rate, the studies revisited have explored both its indirect and direct consequences upon body weight, food intake, hypothalamic function, adipoinsular axis activity, and the

• Address all correspondence to: Eduardo Spinedi, PhD. Neuroendocrine Unit, IMBICE. PO Box 403, 1900 La Plata, Argentina. FAX: +54.221.4253320. E-mail: spinedi@imbice.org.ar
+, Deceased on November 17, 2011.

sensitivity of various tissues to insulin and leptin stimuli. The role of the AT dysfunction generated after feeding individuals with a FRD has also been deeply examined. Data collected clearly indicate that the intake of a FRD triggers the development of several features similar to those found in the human phenotype of MS, e.g., hyperadiposity, impaired glucose tolerance, dyslipemia, insulin- and leptin-resistance, enhanced prothrombotic risk and dysfunction of the hypothalamic satiety signal. Moreover, the intake of this diet negatively affects several of the above mentioned functions regardless of whether this interventional diet is applied directly or indirectly and earlier or later to an organism over development. This evidence must help health policy makers to develop/implement appropriate strategies to promote healthy dietary habits in the general population to prevent the development of chronic diseases such as obesity and T2DM, thus improving the population life quality and decreasing the heavy load of these diseases upon health care budgets and society overall.

Keywords: Adipose tissue function, adipokines, lipid composition, oxidative stress, insulin-resistance, leptin-resistance

1. Introduction

Obesity epidemic is a major problem for worldwide health system with a marked increase in childhood [4, 5]. Obesity increases the risk of developing other chronic disorders such as, type 2 diabetes (T2DM), dyslipidemia, metabolic syndrome (MS) and cardiovascular disease [1-3]. Genes and environment play together an important role in the control of normal metabolic-endocrine functions and neuronal development of the new offspring. Since weight and height are highly inheritable traits [6], we need to consider that environmentally-driven changes in body weight occur and genetic factors could increase the susceptibility to environment-facilitated early weight gain [7].

Administration of unhealthy diets to mothers during gestation [8] and/or the early postnatal [9] periods has shown that nutrient restriction, low-protein diets and high-fat/-carbohydrate diets effectively contribute to the development of obesity and T2DM in their offspring [10-12].

Food intake and body weight gain are processes regulated by hypothalamic neurons that are not fully differentiated during the rodent suckling period; thus, an altered nutritional status during this period severely impacts on normal neuron development [13]. In fact, maternal dietary manipulation (e.g. under-/over-nourished mothers) induces a distorted activity of the hypothalamic circuitry that controls appetite in the offspring [14-16]. This circuit involves orexigenic [e.g. neuropetide Y (NPY), agouti-related protein (AgRP)] and anorexigenic [e.g. corticotropin-releasing hormone (CRH), thyrotropin-releasing hormone (TRH), cocaine- and amphetamine-regulated transcript (CART), pro-opiomelanocortin (POMC)] pathways, contributing to maintain energy homeostasis [17]. Carbohydrate-rich diets (mainly sucrose and fructose) have been frequently used to study this issue; although fructose lacks of any short-term stimulatory effect on insulin and leptin production [18], its excessive consumption without appropriate pancreatic and adipose tissue (AT) responses could lead to long-term detrimental effects upon the regulation of energy intake and body adiposity. Nowadays, the *per capita* fructose intake (sucrose- and high-fructose corn syrup-derived) has risen from 64 g/day (during the 70's) to 81 g/day (in the year 1997); an additional fructose intake (2.5

g/day) results from the increased consumption of fruits and vegetables [18]. It has been claimed that such fructose overload leads to an enhanced prevalence of obesity, T2DM and MS [10-12, 19].

It has been reported that offspring born from mothers fed with a fructose-rich diet (FRD) during pregnancy and lactation had decreased body weight, hyperinsulinemia and hypoglycemia at weaning [20]. Moreover, rat pups consuming high-carbohydrate milk during lactation did develop obesity in adulthood [21]. Also, rat offspring consuming fructose-rich milk during the suckling period are characterized by increased body weight, enhanced insulinemia and augmented skeletal muscle fatty acid transport in adult life [22]. Excessive insulin secretion in turn promotes key features such as enhanced lipogenesis [23] and adipogenesis [24], impairs hypothalamic leptin signaling [25] and reduces vagus tone inhibition [26], thus resulting in additional vagus-stimulated insulin secretion [26]. The mechanisms whereby the FRD induces the MS are still, however, not fully understood.

It has been suggested that one of the main mechanisms triggered by the intake of a FRD is an increased production of reactive oxygen species (ROS) that cause oxidative stress (OS) [27]. Whatever the FRD-induced impaired functions are, its intake even for a short period of time settles a vicious circle that assures the persistence of several physiopathological mechanisms that will favor the development of metabolic and cardiovascular disorders.

The aim of this chapter is to recapitulate evidence on the consequences of the intake of a FRD upon: a) changes in the hypothalamic controlling appetite/satiety circuit, several metabolic-endocrine functions (including that of the retroperitoneal adipose tissue; RPAT) of adult male rats born from a primipara mother fed this diet throughout the lactating period, and b) the role played by OS upon the development of abdominal adipose tissue (AAT) dysfunction in normal adult male rats fed with a FRD.

2. Materials and Methods

2.1. Experimental Design I: Impact of FRD Consumption by the Lactating Mother on Metabolic and Neuroendocrine Functions in the First Male Offspring in the Adult Age

2.1.1. Animals and Diets

Sprague-Dawley rats bred in our Institutions were maintained under controlled conditions of temperature (21 ± 2° C) and light (on between 07:00 and 19:00 h) with free access to standard commercial rat chow and water. Virgin females were mated with males in 10 x 20-inch plastic cages (at a 3:1 relation) until positive detection of sperm in their vaginal smears (examined every day at 08:00 h). Pregnant dams were then individually housed in plastic cages, and fed with standard chow and water *ad libitum* throughout pregnancy. Immediately after delivery, litter number was adjusted to 8 pups per dam (average of male pups per litter ranged between 60-65%, approximately). Lactating mothers (LM) with their offspring, fed with standard Purina chow *ad libitum*, were allocated into two groups: one drank tap water (control diet, CD-LM; n = 7), while the other had 10% fructose (w/v) in the drinking water (FRD-LM; n = 8). Fresh fructose solution was provided every 2 days. Mother body weight (BW) and food and fluid intake were recorded every 48 h during lactation. Immediately after weaning, mothers were sacrificed and plasma samples were stored (- 20° C) for measurement of different metabolites. Weaned (21 days of age) male pups (raised from CD-LM and FRD-LM: CD and FRD, respectively) were individually housed and fed with standard Purina chow and water *ad libitum* until sacrifice (60 days of age). During this period, individual BW and food intake were recorded every 48 h. In each group we allocated one male rat from each different litter which resulted (unless indicated) in final groups of 7 CD and 8 FRD male rats. Rats were sacrificed by decapitation following the NIH Guidelines for Care and Use of Experimental Animals. Experiments received approval from our Institutional Committee on Animal Experimentation.

2.1.2. Studies Performed in Basal Condition

After sacrificing CD (n = 7) and FRD (n = 8) animals under basal condition (between 08:00 and 09:00 h) trunk blood was collected into EDTA-coated tubes. Tubes were rapidly centrifuged (4° C; 3,000 rpm) and plasma samples were kept frozen (-20° C) until metabolite measurements. Immediately after sacrifice, the medial basal hypothalamus (MBH) was dissected as previously reported [28] (limits: posterior border of the optic chiasm, anterior border of the mamillary bodies, and lateral hypothalamic borders, 3 mm deep, approximately); tissues were kept frozen (-80° C) until total RNA isolation. RPAT pads were aseptically dissected and placed in (previously weighed) sterile Petri dishes containing 10 ml of sterile Krebs-Ringer-MOPS (Sigma Chem. Co. St. Louis, MO; 1 Krebs-Ringer:3 double distilled H_2O:1 MOPS, pH 7.4) medium. Dishes were weighed and fat mass was calculated by the difference between the recorded weights. RPAT pads were either used for cell isolation/incubation and histological studies or kept frozen (-80° C) until total RNA isolation.

2.1.3. Glucose Tolerance Test (GTT)

Plasma glucose and insulin concentration was measured after a glucose injection (2 g/Kg BW; i.v.) in 60 day-old male rats (n = 7 CD and 8 FRD animals), bearing an indwelling i.v. cannulae (implanted in the right jugular vein 48 h before experimentation). On the morning of the experimental day, a small volume of blood was taken from non-fasting rats before (time 0) and, 5, 15, 30, 60 and 90 min after glucose administration [29]; a similar volume of the blood withdrawn was immediately replaced by artificial plasma. Plasma samples were kept frozen (-20° C) until determination of glucose and insulin.

2.1.4. Hypothalamic Sensitivity to Leptin

These protocols are similar to those previously reported [30, 31], with minor modifications. Briefly, CD and FRD male rats were individually caged and fed *ad libitum* with standard rat chow and water. Rats were daily handled (10 min per day, between 16:00 and 17:00 h) for one week prior to the study.

The first test was set up on the experimental day (age, 60 days). Food was withdrawn between 16:00 and 17:00 h. Thereafter, each group of CD and FRD male rats (n = 5-6 rats per treatment group), received a single i.p. injection of either recombinant mouse leptin (1 mg/kg BW) dissolved in sterile normal saline solution (volume injected, 0.4-0.6 mL/rat) or the same volume of vehicle alone at 17:00 h. Immediately after injection, rats got back to their cages having access to a known amount of rat chow. Four hours after treatment (21:00 h), the remaining amount of food in each cage was carefully removed and weighed: 4-h food intake was then calculated.

The second test was performed in overnight fasting rats (age, 60 days). At 08:00-09:00 h on the experimental day, each group of CD and FRD male rats (n = 5-6 rats per treatment group) were i.p. injected with a small volume of either leptin solution (1 mg/Kg BW) or vehicle. Animals were sacrificed 45 min post-treatment and the MBHs were rapidly dissected and kept frozen (-80° C) until total (STAT-3) and phosphorylated (p-STAT-3) signal transducer and activator of transcription-3 were determined by Western Blot.

2.1.5. Morphological Characteristics of the AT

For histological studies, freshly dissected RPAT pads were fixed in 4% paraformaldehyde (in 0.2 M phosphate buffer) at 4° C (maximum 3 days); they were then washed (0.01 M PBS) and immersed in 70 % ethanol (24 h), and finally embedded in paraffin. Four-µm sections were obtained at different levels of the blocks, stained with hematoxylin-eosin and examined with a Nikon light microscope. Quantitative morphometric analysis was performed using a RGB CCD Sony camera together with the Image Pro-Plus 4.0 software (magnification: 10x). For each fat sample, 7 sections and 3 levels were selected (n = 4 animals per group). Systematic random sampling was used to select 15 fields for each section and 2,500 cells per group were examined. Adipocyte diameter and area were measured [32]; cell volume was then calculated ($4/3\pi.r^3$).

2.1.6. Isolation and Incubation of RPAT Cells

Isolated adipocytes from RPAT pads were obtained as previously and extensively described [33, 34]. Isolated adipocytes were diluted to (approximately) 200,000 cells per 900 µL of Krebs-Ringer-MOPS medium, and distributed into 15 mL plastic tubes. Adipocytes were then incubated 45 min at 37° C in 95% air-5% CO_2 atmosphere with either medium alone (concentration 0) or containing insulin (0.1-10 nM, Novo Nordisk Pharma AG, Switzerland) [34]. At the end of incubation, media were carefully aspirated and kept frozen (-20° C) until measurement of leptin concentrations.

2.1.7. Measurement of Peripheral Biomarkers

Circulating glucose (Wiener Argentina Lab.), total proteins (Wiener), total cholesterol (Wiener), triglyceride (TG; Wiener) and free fatty acid (FFA; Randox Laboratories Ltd., UK) levels were measured using commercial kits. Plasma and medium leptin (LEP) concentrations [33] and circulating levels of insulin [35] and corticosterone [19] were determined by specific radioimmunoassays (RIAs) developed in our laboratories. Plasma levels of other adipokines were measured (ELISA) following manufacturer protocols [36] [Linco Research, Cat. # EZRADP-62K for adiponectin (ADIPOQ); American Diagnostica Inc., CT, USA, IMU-CLONE Cat. # 601 for plasminogen activator inhibitor factor-1 (PAI-1); Life Diagnostics, Inc., PA, USA, Cat. # 2210-2 for C-Reactive Protein (CRP); and Amersham, GE Healthcare, UK, cat. # RPN2744 for tumor necrosis factor α (TNFα)].

2.1.8. Tissue RNA Isolation and Real-Time PCR

Total RNA was isolated from MBH and RPAT pads of different groups by the single-step, acid guanidinium isothiocyanate-phenol-chloroform extraction method (Trizol; Invitrogen, Life Tech., USA; cat. # 15596-026). One μg of total RNA was reverse transcripted using random primers (250 ng) and Superscript III Rnase H-Reverse Transcriptase (200 U/HL Invitrogen, Life Tech, USA; cat # 18989-093). Primers applied (shown in alphabetical order in Table 1) were β-actin (ACTB), ADIPOQ, AgRP, CART, CRH, LEP, NPY, *ob*-Rb, POMC and TRH. Two μL of the reverse transcription mix were amplified with QuantiTect Syber Green PCR kit (Qiagen, cat. # 204143) containing 0.5 μM of each specific primer, using LightCycler Detection System (MJ Mini Opticon, Biorad). PCR efficiency was near 1. The cycle threshold (Ct) was measured in separate tubes by duplicate. The identity and purity of the amplified product were checked by electrophoresis on agarose mini-gels, and analysis of the melting curve was carried out at the end of amplification. Values of the differences between Ct were calculated in every sample for each gene of interest as follows: Ct gene of interest-Ct reporter gene. β-actin, whose mRNA levels did not differ between control and test groups, was the reporter gene. Relative changes in the expression level of one specific gene (ΔΔCt) were calculated as ΔCt of the test group minus ΔCt of the control group, and then presented as 2-ΔΔCt.

2.1.9. Medial Basal Hypothalamus: Western Blot Analysis

Briefly, frozen MBHs were homogenized in lysis buffer: RIPA (Santa Cruz Biotechnology), protease inhibitor cocktail (0.35 mg/ml PMSF, 2 μg/ml leupeptin, 2 μg/ml aprotinin) and phosphatase inhibitor cocktail (10 mM sodium fluoride, 20 mM sodium β-glycerophosphate, and 10 mM benzamidine). After lysis (90 min in ice), samples were centrifuged (10,000 x g at 4° C for 10 min) and soluble protein concentrations of the resulting lysates were determined by Lowry. Proteins (50 μg per lane) were resolved by 10% sodium dodecyl sulfate-polyacrylamide gel electrophoresis. Proteins were then transferred onto polyvinylidene fluoride membranes and incubated overnight at 4 °C with specific primary antibodies directed toward the signal transducer and activator of transcription-3 (anti-phosphorylated-STAT-3 or anti-total STAT-3, from Santa Cruz Biotechnology, Inc.) followed by 1-h incubation at room temperature with the secondary antibody (goat anti-rabbit IgG horseradish peroxidase conjugates; Upstate, Millipore). Following membrane washing, immune complexes were revealed using enhanced chemiluminescence reagents (Amersham Life Science). The intensity of bands was quantified (Section Image Software), and the p-STAT-3/total-STAT-3 ratios were calculated.

2.2. Experimental Design II: Impact of FRD Consumption by the Naive Adult Male Rat

2.2.1. Animals and Diets

Normal male Wistar rats (180-200 g BW) were maintained in a temperature-controlled environment (23° C) with a fixed 12-h light/dark cycle and fed for one week (stabilization period) with a standard laboratory rat diet. After that period, rats were divided into two groups: one was fed with a commercial standard diet and tap water (CD group) during 3 weeks, while the other received the same diet with the addition of 10% fructose (w/v) into the drinking water (FRD group). Fresh fructose solution was daily provided. International regulations concerning the ethical use of animals were followed.

Table 1. Primers used (designed for a high homology region of different genes) for real time RT-PCR. (se: sense; as: anti-sense; GBAN: GenBank Accession Number; amplicon length, in bp)

		GBAN	bp
ACTB	se, 5´-AGCCATGTACGTAGCCATCC-3´	NM_031144	115
	as, 5´-ACCCTCATAGATGGGCACAG-3´		
ADIPOQ	se, 5'-AATCCTGCCCAGTCATGAAG-3'	NM_144744	159
	as, 5'-TCTCCAGGAGTGCCATCTCT-3'		
AgRP	se, 5'-GGGCGTGGCACCACTGAAGG-3'	NM_033650	183
	as, 5'-ACACAGCGACGCGGAGAACG-3'		
CART	se, 5'-AAGGCGGCAACTTCGGGCTC-3'	NM_017110	167
	as, 5'-CGATCCTGGCCCCTTTCCGC-3'		
CRH	se, 5´-GCTAACTTTTTCCGCGTGTT -3´	NM_031019	175
	as, 5´-GGTGGAAGGTGAGATCCAGA-3´		
IRS-1	se, 5´-ACGGTTTCAGAGCAGAGGAA-3´	NM 012969	176
	as, 5´-TGTGCCAAGCAACAAGAAAG-3´		
IRS-2	se, 5´-CCAGGGATGAAGCAGGACTA-3´	AF08764	151
	as, 5´-CTACCCACTGAGCCCAAGAG-3´		
LEP	se, 5´-GAGACCTCCTCCATCTGCTG-3´	NM_013076	192
	as, 5´-CTCAGCATTCAGGGCTAAGG-3'		
NPY	se, 5´-TACTCCGCTCTGCGACACTA-3'	NM_012614	115
	as, 5´-GGGCATTTTCTGTGCTTTCT -3´		
ob-Rb	se, 5´-TGTGGAATCTGGAGTGGTCA -3´	AF287268	115
	as, 5´-TCTGGAGCCTGAACCAGTTT -3´		
POMC	se, 5´-CCTATCGGGTGGAGCACTT-3´	NM_139326	123
	as, 5´-TCTTGATGATGGCGTTCTTG-3´		
TRH	se, 5'-GGGACCTCCTCAGAAAGGAAGGGT-3'	NM_013046	165
	as, 5'-CCCCCACCCCAAGGACATATCTAA-3'		

2.2.2. Chemicals

Standards for HPLC [oxidized and reduced glutathione, α-tocopherol, NAD^+, NADH(H), NADPH(H), thiobarbituric acid, CoA, N-ethylmaleimide, organic and inorganic components for buffer preparations, teraetoxypropane and butylated hydroxytoluene] were purchased from Sigma Chemical Co (St. Louis, Mo, USA). All solvents were HPLC-grade and provided by Carlo Erba (Milano, Italy). Lipid standards for c-gas liquid chromatography (c-GLC) identification were from Serdary Research Laboratories (London, Ontario, Canada). All standards were stored in appropriate solvents under N_2 atmosphere at -20°C. Concentrations and purities were routinely checked by HPLC and/or c-GLC. Other chemicals used were reagent grade and obtained from local commercial sources.

2.2.3. Peripheral Metabolite Measurements

Non-fasting animals were sacrificed and trunk blood was collected into EDTA-coated tubes. Tubes were rapidly centrifuged (4° C at 3000 rpm) and plasma samples immediately analyzed or stored at –20ºC. Plasma glucose, triglyceride and FFA levels were measured using enzymatic commercial kits implemented in an automated clinical analyzer. Plasma insulin concentrations were measured by RIA using an antibody against rat insulin, rat insulin standard (both from Linco Research Inc., IN, USA), and highly purified porcine insulin labeled with ^{125}I [35]. Leptin plasma levels, media concentrations and circulating corticosterone concentrations were measured by previously described and validated RIAs [19]. Circulating levels of other adipokines (ADIPOQ and PAI-1) were measured by commercial kits as mentioned in section 2.1.7.

2.2.4. Glucose Tolerance Test (GTT)

The GTT was performed in 12 h-fasting rats by i.p. injection of a glucose solution (1 g/kg BW in sterile saline solution) [37]. Heparinized blood samples were obtained from the retro-orbital plexus under pentobarbital anesthesia (i.p., 48 mg/kg BW) before and 15, 30, 60 and 120 min after the glucose load. Plasma glucose levels were immediately measured as indicated above.

2.2.5. Histological Studies in AAT

Pieces of AAT were quickly removed after animal killing, immediately fixed in Bouin's fluid and embedded in paraffin. Sections of 4 μm were obtained thereafter at different levels of the blocks and stained with hematoxylin-eosin. In these sections we measured adipocyte diameter and volume [32].

2.2.6. Enzymatic Antioxidant Activities and Lipid Soluble Antioxidants in AAT

Pre-weighed ATT pads were sonicated in buffer containing 50 mM Tris-HCl (pH 7.4), 1.15% KCl, 1 mM N-ethylmaleimide and 0.1 % BHT (v/v), and then centrifuged at 4° C (600 x g). Supernatants were stored at -70ºC under argon atmosphere. Contents of glutathione disulfide (GSSG) were determined by HPLC, while reduced glutathione (GSH) was measured as previously described [37]. Samples for GSSG analyses were obtained in the presence of N-ethylmaleimide, and deproteinized using trichloroacetic acid (15% final concentration). α-tocopherol was determined by HPLC. Cytosolic (Cu, Zn)- and mitochondrial (Mn)-SOD activities were assayed as described earlier [37].

2.2.7. Thiobarbituric acid Reactive Substances (TBARS) Measurement

Frozen pre-weighed AAT pads and plasma samples were processed for measurement of TBARS concentrations. AAT pads were homogenized in a phosphate-buffered solution (pH 7.4) containing 10% KCl; homogenates were stored at -70° C until processed. The extent of lipid peroxidation was determined by measuring TBARS [37]. The amount of TBARS formed was calculated using the extinction coefficient for the malondialdehyde-TBA complex of 1.56×10^5 $(mol/L)^{-1.\ cm-1}$, and expressed as nmol of TBARS per milligram of homogenate protein (Bio-Rad Protein Assay, Rc, USA).

2.2.8. Lipid Composition in AAT

Appropriate aliquots of the incubation media or tissue homogenates were processed by c-GLC analysis. Total lipids were extracted as described elsewhere [37]. c-GLC of the fatty acid methyl esters (FAME) was performed as previously reported [37], except that in this case we used a capillary column (Supelco, Avondale, PA, USA) mounted on a Hewlett Packard HP 6890 Series GC System Plus (Avondale, PA), equipped with a terminal computer integrator system. FAME were identified by comparison of their relative retention times with authentic standards, and mass distribution was calculated electronically by quantification of the peak areas.

2.2.9. Leptin Release by AAT

A few milligrams of pre-weighed AAT pads were incubated for 120 min at 37° C in Krebs-Ringer-bicarbonate buffer, pH 7.4, previously gassed (5% CO_2-95 b% O_2). FFA released into the media were then measured as already described [37]. Isolated adipocytes from pre-weighed AAT pads were obtained as previously described [33, 34]. Briefly, fat pads were transferred into sterile plastic tubes containing 4 ml/g fat of Krebs-Ringer-MOPS medium with 1 g % w/v of BSA, antibiotics, and supplemented with 1 mg/ml collagenase type 1 (Sigma) (pH 7.4). Tubes were incubated at 37° C with gentle shaking for 40 min. Fat suspension was filtered through a nylon cloth and centrifuged (30 sec at 400 rpm) at room temperature. Infranatants were aspirated, and adipocytes were washed with 10 ml of fresh sterile Krebs-Ringer-MOPS-BSA medium and centrifuged as described above (3 times). After washing, cells were diluted with sterile Dulbeccos's Modified Eagle's Medium (Sigma) [supplemented with 1 g % w/v of BSA (Sigma), 1% v/v of FCS and antibiotics, pH 7.4, (Incubation Medium] in order to obtain (approximately) 200,000 adipocytes per 900 μl of medium. Cells were distributed (200,000 cells per tube) in 15 mL conical tubes. The substances tested (diluted in 100 μl) were incubation medium either alone (basal) or containing insulin (0.1-10 nM, Novo Nordisk Pharma AG, Switzerland) or dexamethasone (DXM; 25-100 mM) [34]. Adipocytes were then incubated for 45 min at 37° C in a 95% air-5% CO_2 atmosphere. Each condition was run in five replicates per experiment, and 3-4 different experiments were performed. At the end of incubations, media were carefully aspirated and kept frozen (-20° C) until measurement of leptin concentrations.

2.2.10. Gene Expression in AAT

Total RNA was isolated from AAT pads of both (CD and FRD male rats) groups as mentioned in 2.1.8. For quantitative real-time PCR, the primers used are also shown in Table 1, and the steps followed to perform the calculations of gene expression are similar to those described above (see 2.1.8). Values of the differences between the Ct were calculated in every sample for each gene of interest as follows: Ct gene of interest-Ct reporter gene. β-actin, whose mRNA levels did not differ between control and test groups, was the reporter gene. Relative changes in the expression level of one specific gene (ΔΔCt) were calculated as ΔCt of the test group minus ΔCt of the control group, and then presented as 2-ΔΔCt.

3. STATISTICAL ANALYSIS

All data have been expressed as mean values (± SEM). Data were analyzed by ANOVA (one- or two-factor) followed by post-hoc comparisons with Fisher's test. The areas under the curves of glucose values during the high glucose load test were calculated and analyzed as previously reported [37]. Morphometric data were analyzed by the Least Significant Difference test for multiple comparisons [36]. The nonparametric Mann-Whitney test was used to analyze data from AT mRNA expression and those emerged from Western-blot studies [38]. P values resulting lower than 0.05 were considered as evidence for statistical significance.

4. RESULTS

4.1. Experiment 1: FRD Administration to Normal Lactating Mothers: Neuroendocrine and Metabolic Impact on the First Adult Male Offspring

4.1.1. Body Weight, Energy Intake and Peripheral Metabolites in Lactating Mothers

Similar BW was recorded in mothers from both groups at the beginning and at the end of the lactation period (Table 2). No measurable differences between groups were recorded in the average 48 h-accumulated calorie intake throughout that period (Table 2). At the end of the lactation period, no significant differences in the circulating levels of several metabolites were detected in the CD-LM and FRD-LM groups (Table 2).

4.1.2. Impact of FRD Administration to Lactating Mothers upon Offspring BW, Food Intake and Peripheral Biomarkers

After weaning, male offspring of the FRD group were heavier between 21 and 60 days of age (Figure 1, upper panel). No differences in 48 h-accumulated food intake were observed in individual male pups from both groups at that time-period. Conversely, between days 49 and 60 of age, FRD male pups ate a significantly ($P < 0.05$) larger amount of food than the age-matched CD male rats (Figure 1, lower panel; 27.45 ± 1.11 and 31.49 ± 1.33 g/rat in the last 24 h in CD and FRD groups, respectively; $P < 0.05$).

Sixty day-old male offspring of the two groups displayed similar circulating levels of glucose, triglyceride, total cholesterol, FFAs, total proteins and corticosterone (Table 3). Conversely, FRD male rats had significantly ($P < 0.05$) higher plasma concentrations of insulin than age-matched CD rats (Table 3). These high circulating insulin levels were already observed at 30 days of age, accompanied by a significant decrease in glycemia and an increase in triglyceridemia; these alterations however were no longer recorded at the age of 60 days (data not shown).

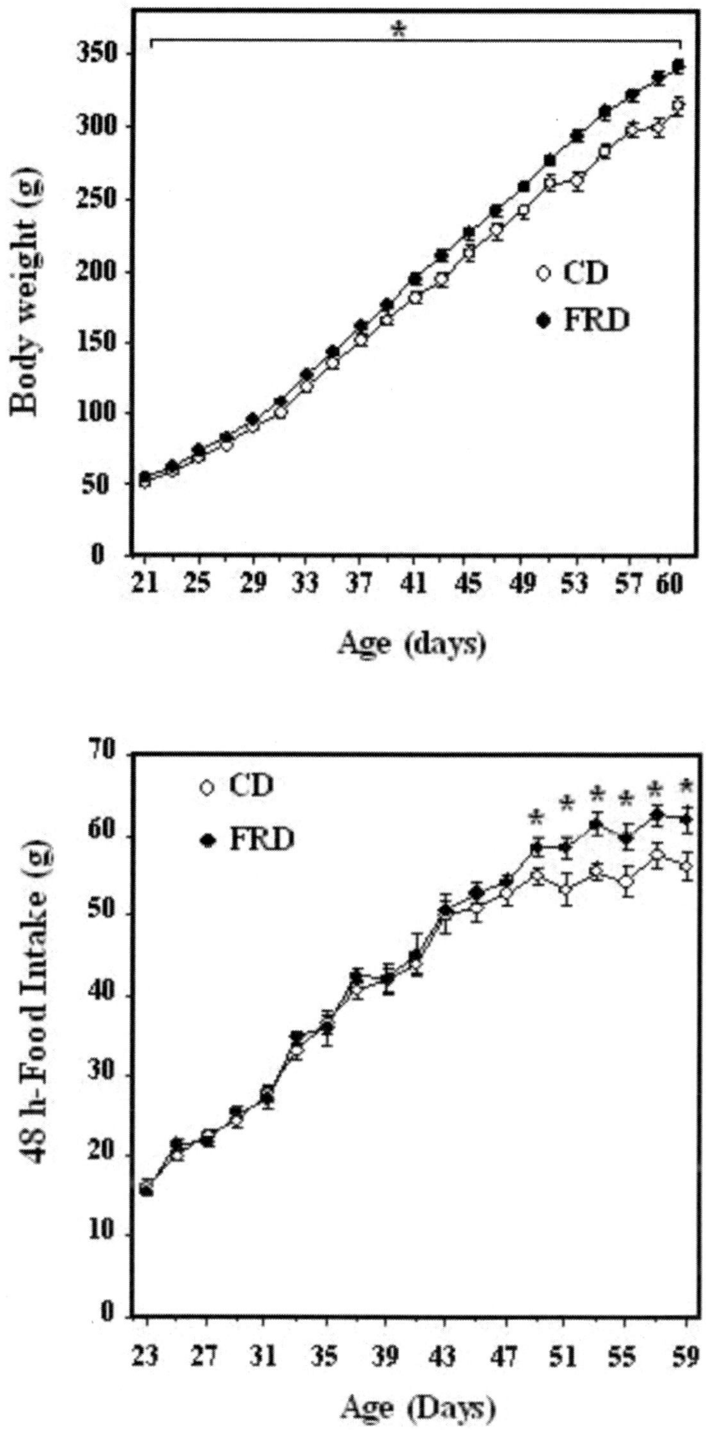

Figure 1. Body weight (upper panel) and 48-h accumulated food intake (lower panel) in CD and FRD male rats after weaning. These parameters were recorded on alternate days of age (between days 21-60 of age for BW and between days 23-59 of age for food intake). Values are means ± SEM (n = 25-30 rats per group, randomly selected from different litter-groups, respectively).
*, $P < 0.05$ vs. CD values on the same day.

Table 2. Changes in BW and average of calorie intake throughout the lactation period in CD-LM and FRD-LM. The circulating levels of several metabolites in mothers from both groups (CD-LM and FRD-LM) evaluated on the weaning day are also shown

	CD-LM	FRD-LM
Initial Body Weight (g)	275.11 ± 6.54	283.19 ± 6.18
Final Body Weight (g)	313.58 ± 13.21	317.72 ± 9.29
Energy Intake (Kj/day)	619.40 ± 41.76	687.22 ± 32.17
Glycemia (mM)	5.69 ± 0.26	5.47 ± 0.35
Triglyceride (mM)	0.44 ± 0.03	0.61 ± 0.06
Total Cholesterol (mM)	1.84 ± 0.10	1.98 ± 0.18
Total Protein (g/L)	10.83 ± 1.32	10.36 ± 0.63
Leptin (ng/mL)	0.82 ± 0.19	0.92 ± 0.25
Corticosterone (nM)	205.79 ± 29.44	170.58 ± 32.89
Insulin (nM)	0.26 ± 0.06	0.31 ± 0.07

Values are means ± SEM (n = 7/8 rats, respectively).

4.1.3. Peripheral Adipokine Profile in 60 Day-old Male CD and FRD Rats

Mothers fed with a FRD throughout the lactation period had significantly ($P < 0.05$) higher and lower circulating levels of leptin and adiponectin, respectively (Table 3). This difference remained even when the serum leptin and adiponectin concentrations were expressed as a function of the individual BW (leptin: 0.79 ± 0.13 and 1.82 ± 0.37 ng LEP/mL/100 g BW; $P < 0.05$; adiponectin: 1.61 ± 0.16 and 1.09 ± 0.07 μg ADIPOQ/mL/100 g BW in CD and FRD rats, respectively, $P < 0.05$). Conversely, comparable plasma levels of other adipokines such as PAI-1, CRP and TNFα, were recorded in both groups of rats, regardless of their BW (Table 3).

Table 3. Basal circulating levels of several metabolites in adult CD and FRD male rats

	CD	FRD
Glucose (mM)	6.60 ± 0.16	6.55 ± 0.22
Triglyceride (mM)	1.44 ± 0.15	1.51 ± 0.16
Total Cholesterol (mM)	1.58 ± 0.08	1.42 ± 0.10
FFAs (mM)	1.05 ± 0.13	1.03 ± 0.12
Total Proteins (g/L)	7.58 ± 0.53	7.29 ± 0.59
Corticosterone (nM)	134.79 ± 31.17	240.09 ± 48.49
Insulin (nM)	0.31 ± 0.02	0.45 ± 0.03*
LEP (ng/mL)	2.41 ± 0.35	6.26 ± 1.56*
ADIPOQ (μg/mL)	5.87 ± 0.66	3.59 ± 0.27*
PAI-1 (ng/mL)	1.44 ± 0.06	1.45 ± 0.18
CRP (mg/mL)	0.36 ± 0.07	0.26 ± 0.22
TNFα (pg/mL)	84.11 ± 0.73	88.93 ± 1.99

Each rat assigned to a group derived from a different litter. Values represent the mean ± SEM. CD (n = 7) and FRD (n = 8) male rats. *, $P < 0.05$ *vs.* CD values.

4.1.4. GTT in Adult Male Offspring from CD or FRD Lactating Mothers

The pattern of circulating glucose levels (Figure 2, panel A) and the area under the curve (AUC) of blood glucose levels (Figure 2, panel B) throughout the i.v.-GTT were similar in the two groups of male rats. Sixty min after glucose administration, blood glucose values had returned to those recorded at basal (sample time 0) in all groups tested.

Conversely, significantly ($P < 0.05$ *vs.* CD values) higher circulating insulin levels were found in FRD male rats on several times throughout the i.v.-GTT (Figure 2, panel C). Moreover, whereas in CD male rats the circulating levels of insulin recorded at 30 min post-glucose load returned to basal, in FRD male rats such recovery was delayed up to 60 min post-glucose load (Figure 2, panel C). Accordingly, the AUC of insulin values was significantly ($P < 0.05$) higher in FRD than in CD male rats (Figure 2, panel D).

4.1.5. Adult Offspring RPAT: Morphological Characteristics and Function

We found that RP fat mass was similar in both groups of male rats (Table 4). However, RP adipocyte diameter, area and volume were significantly ($P < 0.05$) higher in FRD than in CD male rats (Table 4).

The high peripheral levels of leptin measured in FRD male rats correlated well with the LEP mRNA expression in RP fat pads: this parameter was approximately 3.7 times higher ($P < 0.05$) in RP fat pads from FRD than in those from CD male rats (Table 4). Conversely, no group differences were found in RP fat ADIPOQ mRNA expression (Table 4).

Figure 3 shows the results of *in vitro* leptin release by isolated RP fat adipocytes incubated without (spontaneous) or with insulin (0.1-10 nM). Spontaneous leptin output was significantly ($P < 0.05$) higher in adipocytes isolated from RP of the FRD than in those from the CD group. While 0.1 nM insulin did not enhance leptin secretion in either group, 1 and 10 nM insulin significantly ($P < 0.05$) increased leptin release over the baseline only in cells from CD male rats. Conversely, in adipocytes isolated from FRD male rats, insulin significantly enhanced leptin secretion over the respective baseline, only at the highest concentration tested (10 nM) ($P < 0.05$).

Table 4. Retroperitoneal adipose tissue mass, adipocyte characteristics and, leptin (LEP) and adiponectin (ADIPOQ) mRNA expression of adult CD and FRD male rats

	CD	FRD
Pad mass (g/rat)	2.09 ± 0.18	2.05 ± 0.24
Adipocyte diameter (μm)	37.21 ± 0.09	45.45 ± 0.25*
Adipocyte area (μm^2)	1,182.34 ± 10.64	1,807.18 ± 20.29*
Adipocyte volume ($\mu m^3 x 10^3$)	26.97 ± 1.84	49.18 ± 3.39*
LEP mRNA (AU)	1.09 ± 0.19	3.69 ± 0.85*
ADIPOQ mRNA (AU)	1.27 ± 0.41	2.36 ± 0.62

Each rat assigned to a group derived from a different litter. AU: arbitrary units. Values are means ± SEM. CD (n = 4) and FRD (n = 5) male rats. *, $P < 0.05$ vs. CD values.

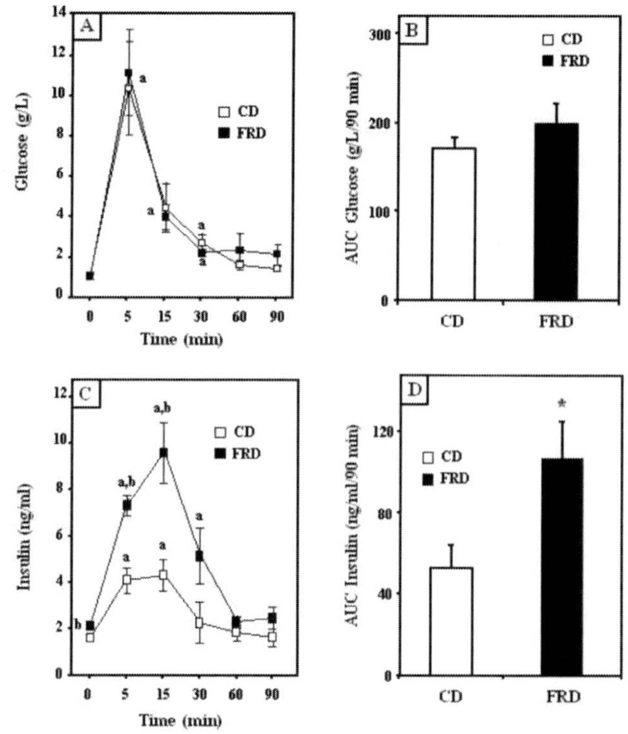

Figure 2. Plasma glucose (panel A) and insulin (panel C) concentrations before (time zero) and after a high glucose load in 60-day-old CD (n = 7) and FRD (n = 8) male rats. Each rat assigned to a group derived from a different litter. The area under the curves (AUC) of glucose and insulin values throughout the GTT in both groups is shown (panels B and D, respectively). Data are means ± SEM.
a, $P < 0.05$ vs. time 0 values in the same group.
b, $P < 0.05$ vs. CD values at same time.
*, $P < 0.05$ vs. CD values.

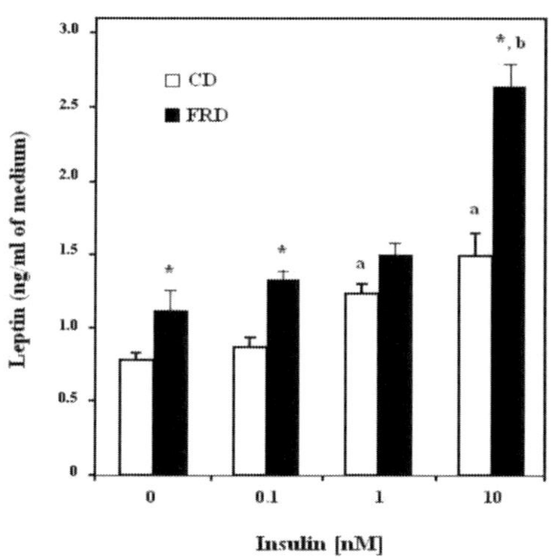

Figure 3. Spontaneous (insulin 0 nM) and insulin (0.1-10 nM)-induced leptin release by isolated RPAT adipocytes obtained from 60 day-old CD and FRD male rats. Data are means ± SEM (n = 3 different experiments using rats from different litters; 5 replicates per condition were run in each experiment).
a, $P < 0.05$ vs. insulin 0 nM values in the CD group.
b, $P < 0.05$ vs. insulin 0 nM values in the in the FRD group.
*, $P < 0.05$ vs. CD values in similar condition.

Table 5. Hypothalamic mRNA expression of genes involved in the local circuitry controlling food intake in adult CD and FRD male rats

	CD	FRD
CRH	1.02 ± 0.12	0.41 ± 0.16 *
TRH	1.01 ± 0.11	0.44 ± 0.09 *
***ob*-Rb**	1.03 ± 0.29	0.27 ± 0.06 *
AgRP	0.99 ± 0.12	1.19 ± 0.11
CART	1.00 ± 0.21	0.62 ± 0.28
NPY	1.01 ± 0.51	0.87 ± 0.23
POMC	1.02 ± 0.33	1.35 ± 0.41

Each rat assigned to a group derived from a different litter. Values are means ± SEM of arbitrary units. CD (n = 4) and FRD (n = 6) male rats. *, P < 0.05 *vs.* CD values.

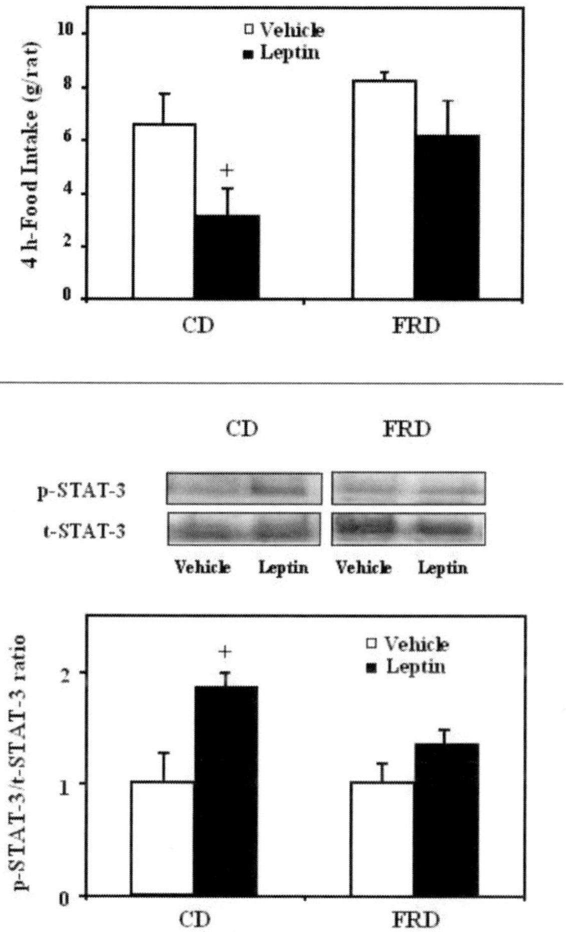

Figure 4. Four-h food intake by adult CD and FRD male rats after either leptin (i.p. 1 mg/Kg BW injection; n = 5 CD and 6 FRD animals) or vehicle (n = 5 CD and 6 FRD animals) treatment (upper panel). In addition, western blot analysis of phosphorylated and total STAT-3 (p- and t-STAT-3, respectively) in hypothalamic protein extracts from fasted 60-day-old CD and FRD male rats, 45 min after i.p. treatment with either vehicle (n = 5 CD and 6 FRD animals) alone or containing leptin (1 mg/Kg BW; n = 5 CTR and 6 FRD animals) is shown (lower panel). Each rat assigned to a group-treatment derived from a different litter. Values are means ± SEM.
+, P < 0.05 vs. vehicle-values.

4.1.6. Hypothalamic Circuitry Controlling Food Intake in Adult Male Rats

Based on the increase in BW (days 21-60 of age) and the daily food intake recorded in FRD male rats at 48-60 days of age, we decided to examine the hypothalamic profile of different appetite-controlling signals. In these animals, the hypothalamic gene expression of CRH, TRH and *ob*-Rb was significantly ($P < 0.05$) lower than in CD male rats (Table 5). Conversely, the hypothalamic mRNA expression of other appetite controlling factors, such as AgRP, CART, NPY and POMC remained at comparable levels in both experimental groups (Table 5).

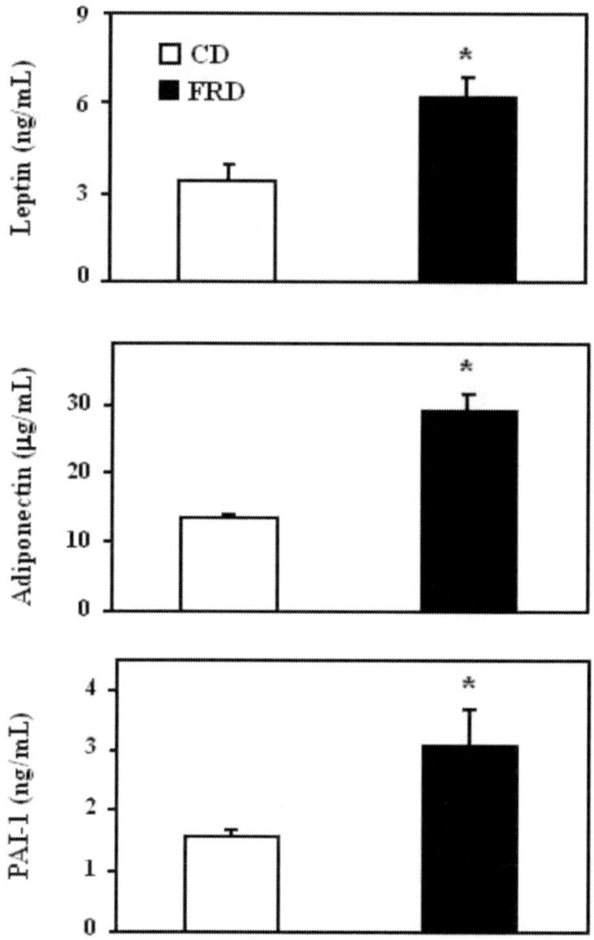

Figure 5. Plasma concentrations of leptin (upper panel), adiponectin (middle panel) and PAI-1 (lower panel) in CD and FRD rats. Values are means ± SEM (n = 6/7 animals per group).
*, $P < 0.05$ vs. CD values.

4.1.7. Leptin Sensitivity in the CD and FRD Offspring

On account of the observed high leptinemia and decreased hypothalamic expression of *ob*-Rb mRNA in adult FRD male rats, we performed two different leptin tests in rats from both experimental groups.

Intraperitoneal injection of leptin (1 mg/kg BW) induced an uneven effect on food intake: it significantly (P < 0.05 *vs.* vehicle-injected CD rats) reduced 4-h food intake in CD male rats but failed to induce any significant change in FRD rats (Figure 4, upper panel).

Additionally, we also measured the effect of the same amount of leptin injection (1 mg/ Kg BW, i.p.) upon STAT-3 phosphorylation in the hypothalamus of fasted rats from the different experimental groups. For that purpose, STAT-3 phosphorylation levels were normalized to total-STAT-3, and value 1 was attributed to the p-STAT-3/total-STAT-3 ratio measured in vehicle-injected animals of the same experimental group (CD and FRD). A significant increase of this ratio in leptin-treated rats was taken as an index of the hypothalamic responsiveness to the hormone. As depicted, while leptin treatment significantly (P < 0.05) increased STAT-3 phosphorylation in CD rats, this effect was absent in FRD rats (Figure 4, lower panel).

4.2. Experiment II: Effect of Short-Time FRD Administration to Naive Adult Male Rats

4.2.1. Dietary Intake, BW and Peripheral Biomarkers in Adult CD and FRD Male Rats

The 21 day-average food intake in CD and FRD animals was 19.2 and 13.3 g/rat/day, respectively. Since FRD rats consumed an average of 5.26 g fructose/rat/day, there was not a significant difference in the daily calorie intake between both experimental groups (55.65 ± 4.54 and 50.79 ± 3.43 Kcal/day, in CD and FRD rats respectively; n = 12/15 rats per group). Moreover, similar BW values were recorded in both experimental groups (initial and final values: 192.3 ± 1.7 and 262.4 ± 2.5 g in CD rats, and 190.7 ± 1.6 and 263.7 ± 2.4 g in FRD rats; n = 12/15 rats per group).

FRD rats displayed significantly (P < 0.05) higher plasma levels of glucose, triglycerides, FFAs and insulin (Table 6), as well as of leptin, adiponectin and PAI-1 (Figure 5). FRD rats also showed significantly (P < 0.05) higher values of both HOMA-R and the AUC of plasma glucose values after a glucose load (Table 6). Finally, no differences in circulating corticosterone levels were found between groups (9.01 ± 2.62 and 8.22 ± 1.45 μg/dl in CD and FRD rats, respectively).

Table 6. Plasma concentration of several biomarkers in CD and FRD rats

	CD	FRD
Glycemia (mM)	7.16 ± 0.27	8.27 ± 0.23*
Triglyceride (mM)	0.76 ± 0.08	1.28 ± 0.07*
FFA (mM)	6.28 ± 0.30	9.43 ± 0.41*
Insulin (ng/mL)	2.69 ± 0.49	4.71 ± 0.61*
HOMA-R	21 ± 3.4	39.9 ± 5.3*
AUC of Glucose**values (mM.min)**	1.56 ± 0.64	4.29 ± 0.49*

AUC: area under the curve. Values are means ± SEM (n = 6/7 animals per group). *, P < 0.05 or less *vs.* CD values.

Table 7. Abdominal adipose tissue (AAT) mass, adipocyte number, diameter and volume

	CD	FRD
AAT Pad Mass (g per rat)	2.46 ± 0.29	1.87 ± 0.21*
Adipocyte number (cells per gram of AAT x 10^6)	2.69 ± 0.21	1.74 ± 0.16*
Adipocyte number (cells per mm^2)	1.81 ± 0.14	1.22 ± 0.11*
Adipocyte diameter (μm)	48.2 ± 2.6	54.1 ± 2.6*
Adipocyte volume (μm^3 x 10^3)	89.57 ± 33.69	119.52 ± 12.83*

Cell counting was performed in 10 fields per section; n = 3 animals per group Values are means ± SEM. *, P < 0.05 or less *vs.* CD values.

4.2.2. FRD-induced Modifications in AAT Mass and Adipocyte Characteristics

The intake of FRD by rats elicited a slight enlargement of AAT mass (2.46 ± 0.29 and 1.87 ± 0.21 g, in FRD and CD rats, respectively; P < 0.05). On the other hand, AAT pads from FRD rats digested with collagenase resulted in a significantly (P < 0.05) lower (vs. CD) number of adipocytes (Table 7). These data fully agree with the morphological characteristics of these cells: AAT adipocytes from FRD rats displayed a significant (P < 0.05 vs. CD cells) increase in their diameter and volume (Table 7).

Table 8. Fatty acid (FA) composition of AAT in CD and FRD rats

FA	CD	FRD
14:0	2.5 ± 0.2	2.8 ± 0.1
16:0	26.8 ± 2.3	29.5 ± 2.0
16:1	1.6 ± 0.1	0.7 ± 0.1*
18:0	16.0 ± 0.7	20.0 ± 0.9*
18:1	15.0 ± 0.5	12.0 ± 0.3*
18:2n-6	12.6 ± 0.4	15.3 ± 0.8*
18:3n-3	0.5 ± 0.05	0.9 ± 0.03*
20:3n-6	0.5 ± 0.03	0.8 ± 0.01*
20:4n-6	24.5 ± 3.3	18.0 ± 3.1
Σ Sat/ Σ Mon	2.73 ± 0.03	4.12 ± 0.07*
Σ PUFA	38.1 ± 0.9	35.0 ± 0.8*
Σ Sat/ Σ PUFA	1.19 ± 0.05	1.49 ± 0.04*

Values are means ± SEM. *, P < 0.05 or less vs. CD values.

Table 9. Relative composition of fatty acid (FA) spontaneously released into the incubation medium by incubated AAT pads from CD and FRD rats

FA	CD	FRD
14:0	2.4 ± 0.1	1.0 ± 0.02*
16:0	26.3 ± 0.5	48.0 ± 2.3*
16:1	3.6 ± 0.05	3.0 ± 0.1*
18:0	22.2 ± 0.8	22.0 ± 1.0
18:1n-9	19.0 ± 0.7	12.5 ± 0.5*
18:1n-7	0.5 ± 0.03	2.0 ± 0.04*
18:2n-6	21.6 ± 1.1	9.0 ± 0.1*
Σ 18:3	1.8 ± 0.1	0.5 ± 0.03*
20:4n-6	2.3 ± 0.1	1.0 ± 0.04*
> PUFA	0.3 ± 0.03	0.5 ± 0.01*
Σ Sat	50.9 ± 1.0	71.0 ± 1.1*
Σ Sat/ Σ Mon	2.20 ± 0.28	4.06 ± 0.26 *
Σ PUFA	56.1 ± 2.0	30.7 ± 1.1 *
Σ Sat/ Σ PUFA	0.91 ± 0.10	2.31 ± 0.23*

Values are means ± SEM (n = 3 experiments, 5 replicates per group). *, P < 0.05 or less vs. CD values.

4.2.3. Impact of FRD on AAT FA Composition/Release and Redox State

The FRD induced marked changes in FA composition of triglycerides from AAT (Table 8). FRD administration for 3 weeks increased significantly (P < 0.05) the proportion of stearic acid (18:0), while its unsaturated derivative, oleic acid (18:1) showed a significant (P < 0.05) 25 % decrease. The polyunsaturated FA (PUFAs) of the n-6 family showed an uneven behavior in rats fed with a FRD: the percentage of linoleic (18:2n-6) and eicosatrienoic (20:3n-6) FAs was increased, the one corresponding to arachidonic (20:4n-6) showed a tendency to diminish and the one of γ-linolenic acid (18:3n-3) was increased. However, the total amount of PUFAs was significantly (P < 0.05) decreased in these rats, with a significant (P < 0.05) increase in the ratios of saturated FA (SFA) to monounsaturated FA (MUFA) and SFA to PUFA (Figure 6, upper panel).

AAT pads from FRD rats released a higher amount of FFAs into the incubation medium than those of CD rats [0.821 ± 0.083 mg FFA/g AAT *vs.* 0.503 ± 0.065 (n = 5); P < 0.05]. The composition of the FAs released by AAT of both experimental groups during the 120-min incubation period was similar to the one recorded in the AAT, with a switch towards the saturated ones (Table 9). Thus, the total estimated amount of PUFAs released by AAT from FRD decreased significantly with respect to CD animals. In agreement with this result, the ratios of total SFA to MUFAs and of total SFAs to PUFAs were significantly higher in the FRD group (Figure 6, lower panel).

The antioxidant defense system of the AAT was significantly affected by FRD administration (Table 10). The activity of total superoxide dismutase (SOD) [Cu-Zn) and (Mn)-isoenzymes] as well as the total content of GSH were significantly (P < 0.05) lower in ATT homogenates of FRD rats.

Consistent with these findings, the concentration of lipid peroxides measured as TBARS was significantly higher (56%) in AAT and plasma samples of FRD rats as compared to CD animals (Table 10).

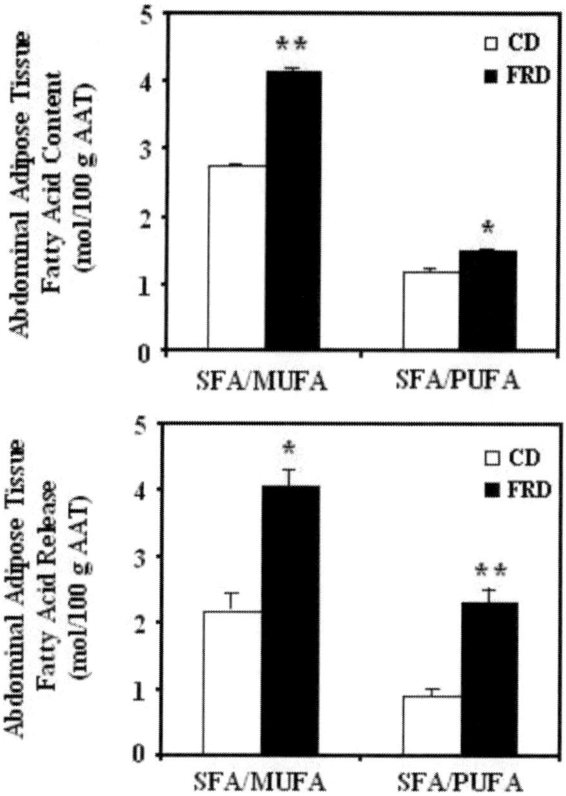

Figure 6. Ratios of saturated (SFA) to monounsaturated fatty acids (MUFA), and SFA to polyunsaturated fatty acids (PUFA) in AAT pads from CD and FRD rats. Upper and lower panels display the ratios in content and release into the medium, respectively. Values are means ± SEM (n = 6 pads per group; 3 different experiments).
*, P < 0.05 or less *vs.* CD values.

Table 10. Changes induced by FRD upon antioxidants enzymes, and OS markers in AAT pads

	CD	FRD
Total SOD (U/mg)	5.93 ± 0.29	3.44 ± 0.17*
(Cu-Zn)-SOD (U/mg)	2.94 ± 0.28	1.26 ± 0.09*
(Mn)-SOD (U/mg)	2.99 ± 0.27	2.17 ± 0.15*
Catalase (U/mg)	0.09 ± 0.01	0.13 ± 0.01*
GSH-Px (U/mg)	2.87 ± 0.08	1.62 ± 0.06*
GSH-TR (U/mg)	12.8 ± 0.24	17.1 ± 0.13*
GSH-R (U/mg)	6.71 ± 0.36	9.62 ± 0.69*
Total GSH (mmol/g)	88.70 ± 3.43	63.90 ± 1.87*
α-Tocopherol (U/mg)	231.01 ± 4.03	135.99 ± 2.04*
β-Carotenoids (U/mg)	0.89 ± 0.02	0.56 ± 0.03
Retinol (U/mg)	0.49 ± 0.03	0.39 ± 0.02*
Lycopenes (U/mg)	0.28 ± 0.02	0.22 ± 0.01*
TBARS (nmol/mg protein)	243.40 ± 12.20	378.91 ± 31.89*

Values are means ± SEM (n = 3 different experiments, 5 replicates per group). *, P < 0.05 or less vs. CD values.

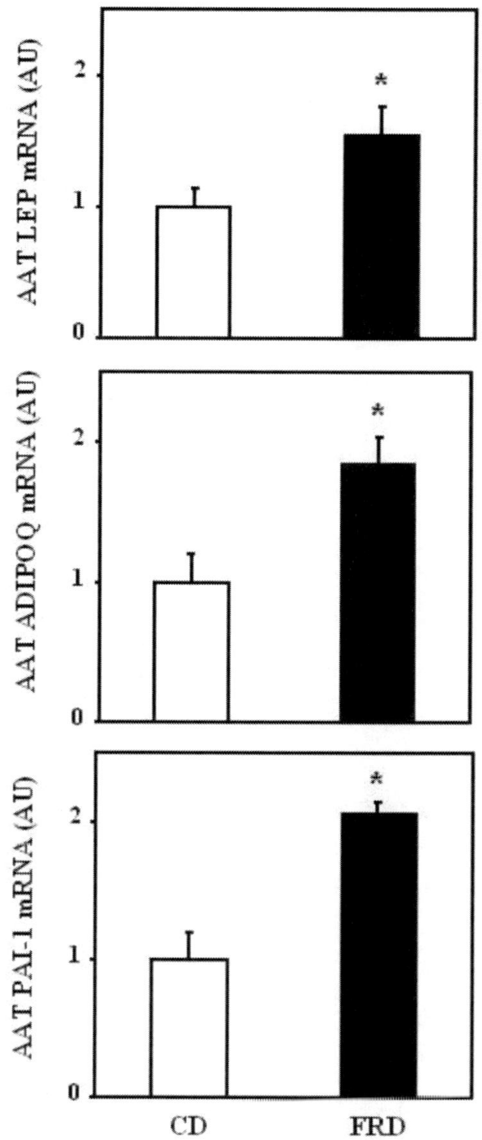

Figure 7. Leptin (LEP), adiponectin (ADIPOQ) and PAI-1 mRNA concentration measured in AAT pads from CD and FRD rats by q-PCR. Data were normalized to the levels of ACTB, and then presented as relative to values obtained in fat pads from CD rats. Values are means ± SEM (n = 3-4 pads per group).
*, $P < 0.05$ vs. CD values.

4.2.4. Adipokines, IRS-1 and IRS-2 mRNAs Expressions in AAT Pads

In agreement with the higher circulating leptin levels and the increased size of adipocytes in the FRD group, the AAT mRNA concentration of various adipokines (LEP, ADIPOQ and PAI-1) was significantly ($P < 0.05$) higher in these rats as compared with CD rats (Figure 7; upper, middle and lower panels, respectively). Conversely, IRS-1 and IRS-2 mRNAs concentrations were significantly lower ($P < 0.05$ *vs.* respective CD values) in AAT pads from FRD rats (Figure 8).

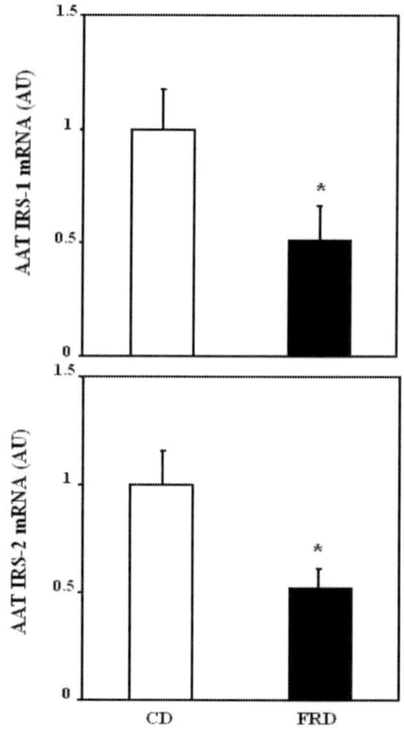

Figure 8. IRS-1 and IRS-2 mRNA expression in AAT pads from CD and FRD rats by q-PCR. Data were normalized to the levels of ACTB, and then presented as relative to values obtained in fat pads from CD rats. Values are means ± SEM (n = 3-4 pads per group). *, $P < 0.05$ vs. CD values.

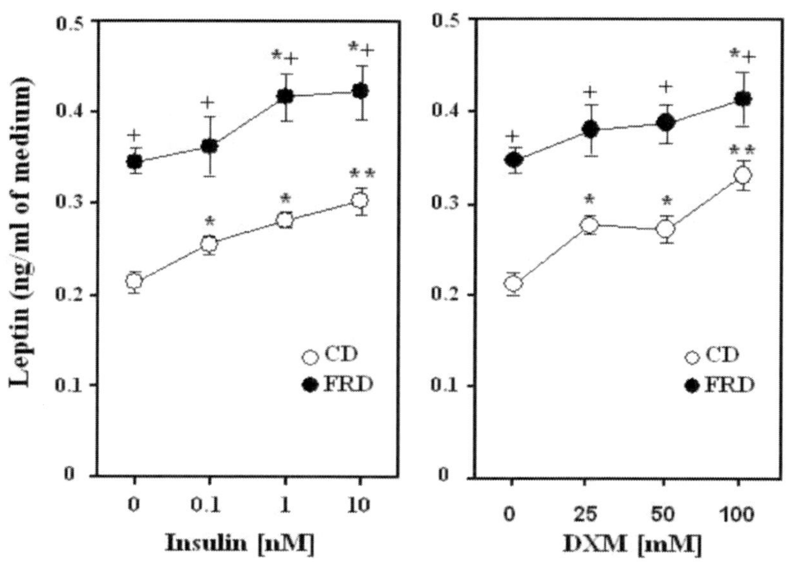

Figure 9. Effects of increasing concentrations of insulin (left panel) and dexamethasone (DXM) (right panel) on leptin release by adipocytes isolated from AAT of CD and FRD rats.
Values represents means ± SEM (n = 4-5 different experiments).
*, $P < 0.05$ *vs.* respective 0 nM insulin/dexamethasone values.
**, $P < 0.05$ *vs.* insulin 0 and 0.1 nM values.
+, $P < 0.05$ *vs.* CD values under similar conditions.

4.2.5. In Vitro Leptin Secretion by Isolated Adipocytes from CD and FRD Rats

Coincident with the data of gene LEP expression in adipocytes of AAT pads from FRD rats, their adipocytes released a significantly ($P < 0.05$) higher amount of leptin than those from CD rats, regardless of the stimulus employed (0.1-10 nM insulin or 25-100 mM dexamethasone; Figure 9 left and right panel, respectively). Insulin-induced leptin secretion exhibited a concentration-dependent profile in both cell-groups (Figure 9, left panel). It should be noted however, that the insulin-induced leptin release was shifted to the right in adipocytes from FRD rats, thus indicating a decreased response to the hormone.

Table 11. *In vitro* leptin-releasing activities of several concentrations of insulin and dexamethasone (DXM) upon isolated AAT adipocytes from CD and FRD rats

		CD	FRD
Insulin (nM)	0.1	1.22	1.04
	1	1.33	1.19
	10	1.44	1.21
DXM (mM)	25	1.31	1.09
	50	1.30	1.13
	100	1.59	1.19

The leptin-release ratio between the concentration measured at a given stimulus concentration and that obtained in its absence was considered 1.00. Data calculated from those depicted in Figure 9 (both panels).

A similar behavior was observed when adipocytes from both groups were incubated with various concentrations of dexamethasone (25-100 mM): adipocytes isolated from FRD animals only secreted a significant ($P < 0.05$ *vs.* stimulus concentration zero) amount of leptin when incubated with the highest dexamethasone concentration (100 mM) (Table 11). Thus, probably FRD broadly affects the stimulus-leptin secretion coupling process and not only a single one mechanism.

5. DISCUSSION

5.1. Detrimental Long-term Effect of Feeding Lactating Mothers with a FRD upon the Offspring's Health

Data from the first set of experiments showed that administration of an iso-caloric FRD to the lactating mother seriously affected several functions in males from the first progeny during adulthood. Adult male offspring displayed a) increased BW and food intake as well as hyperleptinemia, partially due to the disrupted activity of the hypothalamic circuitry responsible for the control of energy balance, b) an overall decreased insulin and leptin sensitivity, and c) impaired AAT function.

Several studies have focused on the effects of high carbohydrate consumption throughout lactation on the offspring's metabolism, maintaining the same diet in pups [22, 39]. Other researchers have only used dietary manipulation on lactating mothers but, as we also did, feeding the offspring with a standard normal diet. These authors reported: i) smaller male offspring size from mothers fed with a protein-restricted diet [40]; ii) accelerated increase in offspring's BW by reducing the litter number (a pup-overfed model) [41]; and iii) normal offspring's BW when suckled by mothers fed with a high-fat diet [30]. Male offspring of our lactating mothers fed with a FRD exhibited a significant increased BW at 21 to 60 days of age; between 49 to 60 days of age, such increase correlated well with an increase in food intake. These data strongly support that FRD intake by lactating dams induced overweight in their male offspring.

We also found, as other authors did, that the adult male offspring suckled by FRD lactating dams displayed higher insulin levels, without changes in peripheral glucose levels or peripheral lipid profile [20, 39]. Although sucrose consumption during gestation and lactation did not modify the lipid profile, it increased the liver triglyceride content [39]. Conversely, offspring nursed with carbohydrate-rich artificial milk had no changes in the circulating levels of triglycerides [22, 42] or free fatty acids [42], despite an increased rate of lipogenesis [43]. Therefore, although we did not currently evaluate changes in the lipogenic process [e.g. due to FRD-induced OS [44]], its potential role in our FRD male rat model could not be ruled out.

Even though with variations in diet administration, other studies have also reported hyperinsulinemic offspring [21, 45-48]. The cause of the incremented insulin levels could be due to changes in either β-cell function or peripheral insulin sensitivity, or both. In this regard, some authors found a profound impact on the offspring's pancreatic function when pups consumed a carbohydrate-rich diet during the pre-weaning period [49, 50]. Our data clearly indicate that the hyperinsulinemia present in male offspring would be an adaptive role to maintain carbohydrate metabolism within normal range. They also showed that decreased adiponectin and increased leptin serum levels characterized our adult FRD male rats, whereas other adipokines remained unchanged.

Although obesity has been considered a state of chronic inflammation in which several peripheral adipocytokines contribute to impair insulin sensitivity [51], the current data suggest that in our FRD model TNFα (unchanged values) would not participate in the mechanism responsible for such an effect. It is accepted that adiponectin enhances insulin sensitivity [52], while leptin would just have the opposite effect [53, 54]. Thus, the high leptin and low adiponectin serum levels currently measured could contribute to the decreased insulin sensitivity present in our FRD male rats.

The large size of adipocytes from RPAT associated to the enhanced LEP gene expression measured in FRD rats indicates an increased LEP production [55]. Supporting this concept, retroperitoneal adipocytes from FRD rats spontaneously released more leptin than those from CD rats and also displayed an impaired response to insulin stimulation. Since these changes occurred without any significant change in retroperitoneal fat mass, it could be assumed that a modified adipogenic process could take place in adult male offspring nursed by FRD lactating dams; further studies are necessary to support this assumption. It should also be considered that other adipokines might be involved in the FRD-induced adipocyte dysfunction in the male offspring of lactating mothers fed with the FRD [56].

Male offspring of rats fed with a FRD during the lactating period increased their food intake at the age of 49 days and older. On the other hand, consumption of a carbohydrate-rich diet by pups between the 4 and 24 postnatal days increased orexigenic and decreased anorexigenic signals at the hypothalamic level [45]; on due time, these changes would decrease insulin sensitivity. It thus might be possible that the currently recorded significant changes in hypothalamic gene expression of several factors involved in the control of food intake and the modest hyperphagia observed during adulthood in the male offspring nursed by FRD lactating mothers depend on a weaker satiety signaling. Further, the decreased hypothalamic *ob*-Rb gene expression and STAT-3 phosphorylation in response to leptin together with the high circulating levels of leptin recorded in our FRD male rats clearly indicate the presence of a hypothalamic leptin-resistance [58] in these rats. On the other hand, in these animals the down-regulated hypothalamic *ob*-Rb gene expression coexists with an impaired function of the CRH- and TRH-ergic mechanisms [main paraventricular nucleus-derived anorexigenic signals [46]. This fact however, does not discard that other signals of the same origin and with a similar activity [59] could also be involved in the FRD-induced alteration present in adult male offspring. Conversely, the unchanged levels of other hypothalamic factors controlling food intake (mainly from arcuate nucleus origin), such as AgRP, CART, NPY and POMC recorded in our FRD male rats, suggest that they would not play a significant role in the development of an altered appetite control.

Only a few experimental models have studied the consequences of a single nutritional manipulation in mothers during lactation. Earlier reports indicate that as a result of drastic litter size reduction, overfed pups developed hyperinsulinemia, hyperleptinemia and obesity in the adult age [55], without changes in hypothalamic NPY [60]. Others have shown, however, that isolated hypothalamic neurons from overfed pups displayed abnormal responses to several stimuli, underlining the relevance of the impact of overfeeding [61, 62] during lactation and the quality of milk [63] on pups' neuron development.

5.2. FRD Administration to Adult Rats and Adiposity Dysfunction

Data from the second set of experiments showed that administration of a FRD to normal male rats for 3 weeks increases the circulating levels of glucose, triglycerides and FFAs [37]. These changes were associated with a significant increase of serum leptin, adiponectin and PAI-1 levels. No changes were recorded in total cholesterol, C-Reactive Protein or the corticoadrenal hormones. This metabolic and endocrine profile presents most of the characteristics of the human MS [64] and strongly indicates a switch of a selective set of biomarkers from the homeostatic to the allostatic regimen.

Among the abnormal changes identified in FRD rats, we found: a) a significant increase in AAT mass and its adipocyte size, b) a significantly decreased gene expression of IRS1 and IRS2 together with a higher AAT gene expression of LEP, ADIPOQ and PAI-1, c) an increased release of leptin from adipocytes isolated from AAT, and d) a shift to the right in the *in vitro* concentration-response curve of insulin/dexamethasone-stimulated leptin release. This lower sensitivity to the stimulatory effect of insulin on leptin release and the lower expression of IRS-1 and IRS-2 clearly indicate that this tissue plays an active role in the insulin resistant state observed in our FRD rats [37, 65, 66].

On the other hand, our data show that FRD rats have a clear alteration of the AAT endocrine function: there is a significant increase in the peripheral concentrations of leptin and adiponectin, and of several adipokine mRNAs levels in AAT. These adipocytes release a greater amount of leptin in both basal and stimulated (insulin/DXM) conditions. All these changes could be ascribed to the larger adipocyte size measured in these animals and to their increased expression of the LEP mRNA [55]. On due time, the high leptin production could contribute to impair adipocyte response to insulin by affecting both the hormone binding to its receptor [53] and the expression of the downstream receptor mediators IRS-1 and IRS-2 [54, 67].

FRD rats displayed high circulating levels of both insulin and adiponectin, similar to the hormone pattern previously observed in human beings with defective insulin receptor function [68] and in mice with selective inactivation of the insulin receptor gene in their adipocytes [69]. Since adiponectin enhances insulin sensitivity [52] and FA oxidation [70], its increase in animals with insulin resistance (such as the FRD rats) could represent a compensatory autocrine mechanism to counteract the impaired insulin sensitivity [71]. Regarding the high PAI-1, its production has been associated with enhanced OS [72], enlarged adipocyte size and increased lipid content [72]. Since these latter alterations are present in our FRD rats, they could partly explain their PAI-1 overproduction.

The combined increase in plasma glucose and TG levels in FRD rats currently observed could account for the enhancement in OS in AAT and other tissues [37]. The glucose-induced OS could be ascribed to several mechanisms, namely, damaged antioxidant defense system, increased ROS production, glucose autoxidation [73], nonenzymatic glycosilation [74], and oxidative glycosilation [75]. Our data support previous reports showing that carbohydrate-rich diets did induce a systemic ROS increase [71-82].

The increased AAT TBARS concentration measured in FRD rats could contribute to a systemic increase in OS and to a dysregulation in adipokine production. In fact, our data show that in the AAT of the FRD-fed rats there was an alteration of several OS markers, such as a general decrease in antioxidants and in both the lipophilic (α-tocopherol, β-carotene, retinol, and lycopene) and the hydrophilic (glutathione) cellular compartments. Other authors did also report a decrease in α-tocopherol in tissues different from the AAT after a 30-day FRD intake period [81]. The concomitant decrease in the activity of both SOD isoforms and in the total AAT SOD activity recorded in our FRD rats may contribute to an accumulation of superoxide ion, with the consequent enhancement of antioxidant consumption that might induce an increase in catalase (CAT) and GSH-Tr activities. Indeed, several reports demonstrating that both enzymes are induced by OS strongly support this assumption [83-86]. Whereas glutathione peroxidase activity diminished in FRD rats, GSH-Rd increased significantly; both facts are in agreement with those reported by Martín-Gallán et al. in young diabetic patients [87]. These effects could be due to an excess of GSSG, which in turn promoted an increase in GSH-Rd, as previously reported in different tissues from spontaneously hypertensive rats (SHR) fed with a FRD [86]. Induction of CAT activity was also observed in human patients with impaired glucose tolerance or T2DM, but without any significant change in total SOD activity [88]. Another human study reported increased CAT levels in erythrocytes of hyperlipidemic subjects with concomitant T2DM, and significantly decreased SOD [89]. Since the induction of GSH-Px gene [90] was not found in our FRD rats, we can speculate that the increase in CAT and GSH-Rd may represent a reactive compensatory mechanism for decreased GSH-Px activity, thus removing the endogenous hydrogen peroxide to protect biomembrane lipid peroxidation.

The pro-oxidative FRD-induced state was accompanied by marked changes in AAT FA composition, characterized by a significant increase in SFAs at the expense of total MUFAs and PUFAs. Although there is no previous evidence explaining the mechanism whereby OS modifies AAT FA desaturase activity, our data suggest a blockade in linoleic acid utilization in the n-6 metabolic pathway, leading to arachidonate biosynthesis. Alternatively, the oxidative damage could be the cause for a selective uptake or metabolism of certain FAs, which in turn lead to the AAT fatty acyl alterations. In rats fed with a sucrose-rich diet (SRD) for 6 months, liver desaturase mRNA and biological activities were not affected, but coincidently, such a diet modified the FA composition of serum and liver lipids [91]. However, we cannot discard the possible role of an alteration in the catabolic rate of FAs and/or modifications in their selective uptake and incorporation from the plasma pool in the pathogenesis of these alterations.

AAT from FRD rats released a higher basal amount of FFAs into the medium, suggesting an increase in its lipase activity. Because the AAT is the main source of FFAs for the liver [92], the increased release of FFAs by this tissue together with the IR state would certainly play a key role in the development of hepatic steatosis previously described in rats fed with a FRD [93]. On account of the antilypolitic effect of insulin, we can suggest that the high FFA released by AAT is the consequence of its local IR state. Such assumption is supported by the decreased insulin sensitivity and increased FA and leptin (present study) release from adipocytes obtained in other models fed with high carbohydrate diets for variable periods of time [65, 66, 94]. Moreover, changes in the composition of the FAs released by AAT from FRD rats closely resembled those measured in AAT FA composition. Our results are similar to those reported by Girard et al. in the 16:0, 18:1, 20:4n-6 FAs and total PUFAs in the FA composition of VLDL-LDL lipids of SHR rats fed with a FRD [92]. Indeed, the enhanced OS would also trigger the endocrine AAT dysfunction with a high release of leptin, thus contributing to modify the overall metabolic homeostasis [95].

The impaired glucose tolerance observed in our FRD-fed rats could be a result from at least two abnormal processes measured in these animals: a) the increased ROS production to which pancreatic islet function and β-cell mass are highly sensitive due to their low concentration of antioxidant activity [96], and b) the increased release of FAs, particularly the saturated ones, that exert a deleterious effect upon islet function (lipotoxicity) [97]. Our previous description of the decreased β-cell mass and function induced by administration of a SRD to normal Wistar rats provides a reasonable support to these assumptions [98].

All the FRD-induced changes currently described could be part of an AAT network of interacting abnormalities, namely, the lower insulin antilipolytic effect observed in these rats could be responsible for their high AAT FFAs release and the abnormal pattern of saturated/unsaturated ratio. As mentioned above, the high circulating levels of saturated FFAs could in turn enhance AAT NADPH oxidase activity and ROS production [99]. The increased local ROS production could lead thereafter to the AAT endocrine dysfunction [99]. Indeed, following a similar reasoning, Brownlee et al. have proposed [100] a unifying hypothesis to explain the cause-effect relationship between OS and metabolic/endocrine dysfunctions such as those found in FRD rats. This hypothesis is based on the following: an increased offer of a metabolic substrate will increase ROS mitochondrial production; in turn, enhanced ROS sets off a chain-reaction that a) decreases the antioxidant defense, b) stimulates protein kinase C isoform activity (switching tyrosine to serine-treonine phosphorylation, thus decreasing insulin mediator effectiveness), and c) increases both PAI-1 production and the non-enzymatic glycosylation rate. Thus, it could be assumed that FRD-induced OS at the AAT level could represent a main and early change responsible for most of the metabolic/endocrine abnormalities observed in these animals.

The fact that FRD administration to normal rats induces an increase in serum insulin levels together with an impairment of glucose tolerance suggests that the AAT metabolic/endocrine dysfunction could secondarily affect other tissue functions, such as β-cell insulin secretion. This effect could be ascribed to the deleterious action of both saturated FAs on β-cell function and mass [97], and of ROS due to the low islet antioxidant defense capacity [96].

Conclusion

Our data provide clear objective evidence on the deleterious effect of the intake of unbalanced diets (FRD), comparable to that of the so called ¨modern diets¨. Such an effect could be present after a relatively short period (3 weeks) when administered to adult normal rats, and later in the litters' adulthood when administered to lactating mothers. In fact, we have shown that in lactating mothers the FRD induced neuroendocrine and metabolic derangements in male offspring, which manifested when the progeny reached the adult age. These alterations include a) overweight, b) peripheral tissue resistance to both insulin and leptin associated to high serum levels of these hormones, c) derangement in the hypothalamic circuitry controlling appetite/satiety, and d) large adipocytes with insulin resistance, high leptin expression and secretion. Moreover, when FRD was given to adult naïve male rats, it induced similar alterations together with impaired glucose tolerance and increased AAT content/release of SFAs.

This evidence must alert the population on the deleterious effect of the intake of high-fructose diets either during lactation or in adulthood. It could also prompt public health authorities to define appropriate strategies to develop healthy dietary habits in the general population to prevent the development of diseases related to unhealthy dietary habits. Such policies could decrease the continuous worldwide growth of chronic diseases such as obesity and T2DM, with the consequent improvement in the quality of life of the population, and the heavy load of these diseases upon health care budget and the overall society.

Acknowledgment

Supported by grants from CONICET (PIPs 2009-0704 to ES, and -5020 to JJG) and FONCYT (PICT 2007-1051) of Argentina; and the Fondation pour la Recherche en Endocrinologie (2008/2011; to ES) of Switzerland. ES, JJG and AG are members from the Research Career of CONICET; ORR is member from the La Plata National University Incentives Program.

The authors gratefully thank D. Castrogiovanni and A. Díaz for their commitment with these studies. The edition and correction of the manuscript by Ms. A. Di Maggio is deeply recognized.

REFERENCES

[1] Bray GA, Bellanger T: Epidemiology, trends, and morbidities of obesity and the metabolic syndrome. *Endocrine* 2006;29:109-117.

[2] Reaven G, Abbasi F, McLaughlin T: Obesity, insulin resistance, and cardiovascular disease. *Recent Prog Horm Res* 2004;59:207-223.

[3] Gluckman PD, Hanson MA, Cooper C, Thornburg KL: Effect of in utero and early-life conditions on adult health and disease. *N Engl J Med* 2008;359:61-73.

[4] Rocchini AP: Childhood obesity and a diabetes epidemic. *N Engl J Med* 2002;346:854-855.

[5] Breier BH, Vickers MH, Ikenasio BA, Chan KY, Wong WP: Fetal programming of appetite and obesity. *Mol Cell Endocrinol* 2001;185:73-79.

[6] Barsh GS, Farooqi IS, O'Rahilly S: Genetics of body-weight regulation. *Nature* 2000;404:644–651.

[7] Farooqi S, O'Rahilly S: Genetics of Obesity in Humans. *Endocr Rev* 2006;27:710-718.

[8] Hamilton JK, Odrobina E, Yin J, Hanley AJ, Zinman B, Retnakaran R: Maternal insulin sensitivity during pregnancy predicts infant weight gain and adiposity at 1 year of age. *Obesity* (Silver Spring) 2010;18:340-346.

[9] Patel MS, Srinivasan M: Metabolic programming due to alterations in nutrition in the immediate postnatal period. *J Nutr* 2010;140:658-661.

[10] Taylor PD, Poston L: Developmental programming of obesity in mammals. *Exp Physiol* 2007;92:287-298.

[11] McMillen IC, Robinson JS: Developmental origins of the metabolic syndrome: prediction, plasticity, and programming. *Physiol Rev* 2005;85:571-633.

[12] Plagemann A: Perinatal nutrition and hormone-dependent programming of food intake. *Horm Res* 2006;65(Suppl 3):83-89.

[13] Grove KL, Grayson BE, Glavas MM, Xiao XQ, Smith MS: Development of metabolic systems. *Physiol Behav* 2005;86:646-660.

[14] Plagemann A, Harder T, Melchior K, Rake A, Rohde W, Dörner G: Elevation of hypothalamic neuropeptide Y-neurons in adult offspring of diabetic mother rats. *Neuroreport* 1999;10:3211-3216.

[15] Plagemann A, Harder T, Rake A, Melchior K, Rohde W, Dörner G: Hypothalamic nuclei are malformed in weanling offspring of low protein malnourished rat dams. *J Nutr* 2000;130:2582-2589.

[16] Davidowa H, Plagemann A: Decreased inhibition by leptin of hypothalamic arcuate neurons in neonatally overfed young rats. *Neuroreport* 2000;11:2795-2798.

[17] Schwartz MW, Baskin DG, Kaiyala KJ, Woods SC: Model for the regulation of energy balance and adiposity by the central nervous system. *Am J Clin Nutr* 1999;584:69:584-596.

[18] Elliott SS, Keim NL, Stern JS, Teff K, Havel PJ: Fructose, weight gain, and the insulin resistance syndrome. *Am J Clin Nutr* 2002;76:911-922.

[19] Bray GA, Nielsen SJ, Popkin BM: Consumption of high-fructose corn syrup in beverages may play a role in the epidemic of obesity. *Am J Clin Nutr* 2004;79:537-543.

[20] Rawana S, Clark K, Zhong S, Buison A, Chackunkal S, Jen KL: Low dose fructose ingestion during gestation and lactation affects carbohydrate metabolism in rat dams and their offspring. *J Nutr* 1993;123:2158-2165.

[21] Srinivasan M, Dodds C, Ghanim H, Gao T, Ross PJ, Browne RW, Dandona P, Patel MS: Maternal obesity and fetal programming: effects of a high-carbohydrate nutritional modification in the immediate postnatal life of female rats. Am *J Physiol Endocrinol Metab* 2008;295:E895-E903.

[22] Huynh M, Luiken JJ, Coumans W, Bell RC: Dietary fructose during the suckling period increases body weight and fatty acid uptake into skeletal muscle in adult rats. *Obesity* 2008;16:1755-1762.

[23] Kreier F, Fliers E, Voshol PJ, Van Eden CG, Havekes LM, Kalsbeek A, Van Heijningen CL, Sluiter AA, Mettenleiter TC, Romijn JA, Sauerwein HP, Buijs RM: Selective parasympathetic innervation of subcutaneous and intra-abdominal fat--functional implications. *J Clin Invest* 2002;110:1243-1250.

[24] Gregoire FM, Smas CM, Sul HS: Understanding adipocyte differentiation. *Physiol Rev* 1998;78:783-809.

[25] Münzberg H, Myers MG Jr: Molecular and anatomical determinants of central leptin resistance. *Nat Neurosci* 2005;8:566-570.

[26] Lustig RH: Autonomic dysfunction of the beta-cell and the pathogenesis of obesity. *Rev Endocr Metab Disord* 2003;4:23-32.

[27] Delbosc S, Paizanis E, Magous R, Araiz C, Dimo T, Cristol J-P, Cros G, Azay J: Involvement of oxidative stress and NADPH oxidase activation in the development of cardiovascular complications in a model of insulin resistance, the fructose-fed rat. *Atherosclerosis* 2005;179:43-49.

[28] Spinedi E, Giacomini M, Jacquier MC, Gaillard RC: Changes in the hypothalamo-corticotrope axis after bilateral adrenalectomy: evidence for a median eminence site of glucocorticoid action. *Neuroendocrinology* 1991;53:160-170.

[29] Perelló M, Castrogiovanni D, Moreno G, Gaillard RC, Spinedi E: Neonatal hypothalamic androgenization in the female rat induces changes in peripheral insulin sensitivity and adiposity function at adulthood. *Neuro Endocrinol Lett* 2003;24:241-248.

[30] Niimi M, Sato M, Yokote R, Tada S, Takahara J: Effects of central and peripheral injection of leptin on food intake and on brain Fos expression in the Otsuka Long-Evans Tokushima Fatty rat with hyperleptinaemia. *J Neuroendocrinol* 1999;11:605-611.

[31] Férézou-Viala J, Roy AF, Sérougne C, Gripois D, Parquet M, Bailleux V, Gertler A, Delplanque B, Djiane J, Riottot M, Taouis M: Long-term consequences of maternal high-fat feeding on hypothalamic leptin sensitivity and diet-induced obesity in the offspring. *Am J Physiol Regul Integr Comp Physiol* 2007;293:R1056-R1062.

[32] Moreno G, Perelló M, Camihort G, Luna G, Console G, Gaillard RC, Spinedi E: Impact of transient correction of increased adrenocortical activity in hypothalamo-damaged, hyperadipose female rats. *Int J Obes* 2006;30:73-82.

[33] Giovambattista A, Piermaria J, Suescun MO, Calandra RS, Gaillard RC, Spinedi E: Direct effect of ghrelin on leptin production by cultured rat white adipocytes. *Obesity (Silver Spring)* 2006;14:19-27.

[34] Giovambattista A, Gaillard RC, Spinedi E: Ghrelin gene-related peptides modulate rat white adiposity. *Vitam Horm* 2008;77:171-205.

[35] Perello M, Castrogiovanni D, Giovambattista A, Gaillard RC, Spinedi E: Impairment in insulin sensitivity after early androgenization in the post-pubertal female rat. *Life Sci* 2007;80:1792-1798.

[36] Alzamendi A, Castrogiovanni D, Ortega HH, Gaillard RC, Giovambattista A, Spinedi E: Parametrial adipose tissue and metabolic dysfunctions induced by fructose-rich diet in normal and neonatal-androgenized adult female rats. *Obesity (Silver Spring)* 2009;18:441-448.

[37] Rebolledo OR, Marra CA, Raschia A, Rodriguez S, Gagliardino JJ: Abdominal adipose tissue: early metabolic dysfunction associated to insulin resistance and oxidative stress induced by an unbalanced diet. *Horm Metab Res* 2008;40:794-800.

[38] Zar JH: *Biostatistical Analysis*. Englewood Cliffs. Prentice-Hall, 1974.

[39] Sedová L, Seda O, Kazdová L, Chylíková B, Hamet P, Tremblay J, Kren V, Krenová D: Sucrose feeding during pregnancy and lactation elicits distinct metabolic response in offspring of an inbred genetic model of metabolic syndrome. *Am J Physiol Endocrinol Metab* 2007;292:E1318-E1324.

[40] Zambrano E, Bautista CJ, Deás M, Martínez-Samayoa PM, González-Zamorano M, Ledesma H, Morales J, Larrea F, Nathanielsz PW: A low maternal protein diet during pregnancy and lactation has sex- and window of exposure-specific effects on offspring growth and food intake, glucose metabolism and serum leptin in the rat. *J Physiol* 2006;571:221-230.

[41] Chen H, Simar D, Morris MJ: Hypothalamic neuroendocrine circuitry is programmed by maternal obesity: interaction with postnatal nutritional environment. *PLoS One* 2009;4:e6259.

[42] Aalinkeel R, Srinivasan M, Song F, Patel MS: Programming into adulthood of islet adaptations induced by early nutritional intervention in the rat. *Am J Physiol Endocrinol Metab* 2001;281:E640-E648.

[43] Hiremagalur BK, Vadlamudi S, Johanning GL, Patel MS: Long-term effects of feeding high carbohydrate diet in pre-weaning period by gastrostomy: a new rat model for obesity. *Int J Obes Relat Metab Disord* 1993;17:495-502.

[44] Alzamendi A, Giovambattista A, Raschia A, Madrid V, Gaillard RC, Rebolledo O, Gagliardino JJ, Spinedi E: Fructose-rich diet-induced abdominal adipose tissue endocrine dysfunction in normal male rats. *Endocrine* 2009;35:227-232.

[45] Srinivasan M, Mitrani P, Sadhanandan G, Dodds C, Shbeir-ElDika S, Thamotharan S, Ghanim H, Dandona P, Devaskar SU, Patel MS: A high-carbohydrate diet in the immediate postnatal life of rats induces adaptations predisposing to adult-onset obesity. *J Endocrinol* 2008;197:565-574.

[46] Boullu-Ciocca S, Dutour A, Guillaume V, Achard V, Oliver C, Grino M: Postnatal diet-induced obesity in rats upregulates systemic and adipose tissue glucocorticoid metabolism during development and in adulthood: its relationship with the metabolic syndrome. *Diabetes* 2005;54:197-203.

[47] Fields M, Lewis CG, Lure MD: Responses of insulin to oral glucose and fructose loads in marginally copper-deficient rats fed starch or fructose. *Nutrition* 1996;12:524-528.

[48] Blakely SR, Hallfrisch J, Reiser S, Prather ES: Long-term effects of moderate fructose feeding on glucose tolerance parameters in rats. *J Nutr* 1981;111:307-314.

[49] Vadlamudi S, Hiremagalur BK, Tao L, Kalhan SC, Kalaria RN, Kaung HL, Patel MS: Long-term effects on pancreatic function of feeding a HC formula to rats during the preweaning period. *Am J Physiol* 1993;265:E565-E571.

[50] Aalinkeel R, Srinivasan M, Kalhan SC, Laychock SG, Patel MS: A dietary intervention (high carbohydrate) during the neonatal period causes islet dysfunction in rats. *Am J Physiol* 1999;277:E1061-E1069.

[51] Bastard JP, Maachi M, Lagathu C, Kim MJ, Caron M, Vidal H, Capeau J, Feve B: Recent advances in the relationship between obesity, inflammation, and insulin resistance. *Eur Cytokine Netw* 2006;17:4-12.

[52] Berg AH, Combs TP, Du X, Brownlee M, Scherer PE: The adipocyte-secreted protein Acrp30 enhances hepatic insulin action. *Nat Med* 2001;7:947-953.

[53] Walder K, Filippis A, Clark S, Zimmet P, Collier GR: Leptin inhibits insulin binding in isolated rat adipocytes. *J Endocrinol* 1997;155: R5-R7.

[54] Krempler F, Hell E, Winkler C, Breban D, Patsch W: Plasma leptin levels: interaction of obesity with a common variant of insulin receptor substrate-1. *Arterioscler Thromb Vasc Biol* 1998;18:1686-1690.

[55] Couillard C, Mauriège P, Imbeault P, Prud'homme D, Nadeau A, Tremblay A, Bouchard C, Després JP: Hyperleptinemia is more closely associated with adipose cell hypertrophy than with adipose tissue hyperplasia. *Int J Obes Relat Metab Disord* 2000;24:782-788.

[56] Hirai K, Hussey HJ, Barber MD, Price SA, Tisdale MJ: Biological evaluation of a lipid-mobilizing factor isolated from the urine of cancer patients. *Cancer Res* 1998;58:2359-2365.

[57] Mracek T, Ding Q, Tzanavari T, Kos K, Pinkney J, Wilding J, Trayhurn P, Bing C: The adipokine zinc-alpha2-glycoprotein is downregulated with fat mass expansion in obesity. *Clin Endocrinol (Oxf)* 2010;72:334-341.

[58] Kalra SP, Dube MG, Pu S, Xu B, Horvath TL, Kalra PS: Interacting appetite-regulating pathways in the hypothalamic regulation of body weight. *Endocr Rev* 1999;20:68-100.

[59] Oh-I S, Shimizu H, Satoh T, Okada S, Adachi S, Inoue K, Eguchi H, Yamamoto M, Imaki T, Hashimoto K, Tsuchiya T, Monden T, Horiguchi K, Yamada M, Mori M: Identification of nesfatin-1 as a satiety molecule in the hypothalamus. *Nature* 2006;443:709-712.

[60] Plagemann A, Harder T, Rake A, Waas T, Melchior K, Ziska T, Rohde W, Dörner G: Observations on the orexigenic hypothalamic neuropeptide Y-system in neonatally overfed weanling rats. *J Neuroendocrinol* 1999;11:541-546.

[61] Davidowa H, Li Y, Plagemann A: Altered responses to orexigenic (AGRP, MCH) and anorexigenic (alpha-MSH, CART) neuropeptides of paraventricular hypothalamic neurons in early postnatally overfed rats. *Eur J Neurosci* 2003;18:613-621.

[62] Davidowa H, Plagemann A: Hypothalamic neurons of postnatally overfed, overweight rats respond differentially to corticotropin-releasing hormones. *Neurosci Lett* 2004;16:371:64-68.

[63] Bautista CJ, Boeck L, Larrea F, Nathanielsz PW, Zambrano E: Effects of a maternal low protein isocaloric diet on milk leptin and progeny serum leptin concentration and appetitive behavior in the first 21 days of neonatal life in the rat. *Pediatr Res* 2008;63:358-363.

[64] Grundy SM, Hansen B, Smith SC Jr, Cleeman JI, Kahn RA: Clinical management of metabolic syndrome: report of the American Heart Association/National Heart, Lung, and Blood Institute/American Diabetes Association conference on scientific issues related to management. *Circulation* 2004;109:551-556.

[65] Smith U, Cahlin E, Scherstén T: Sucrose feeding in man. Effects on lipolysis and antilipolytic action of insulin in the adipose tissue. *Acta Med Scand* 1973;194:147-150.

[66] Soria A, D'Alessandro ME, Lombardo YB: Duration of feeding on a sucrose-rich diet determines metabolic and morphological changes in rat adipocytes. *J Appl Physiol* 2001;91:2109-2116.

[67] Cohen B, Novick D, Rubinstein M: Modulation of insulin activities by leptin. *Science* 1996;274:1185-1188.

[68] Semple RK, Soos MA, Luan J, Mitchell CS, Wilson JC, Gurnell M, Cochran EK, Gorden P, Chatterjee VKK, Wareham NJ, O'Rahilly S: Elevated plasma adiponectin in humans with genetically defective insulin receptors. *J Clin Endocrinol Metab* 2006;91:3219-3223.

[69] Blüher M, Michael MD, Peroni OD, Ueki K, Carter N, Kahn BB, Kahn CR: Adipose tissue selective insulin receptor knockout protects against obesity and obesity-related glucose intolerance. *Dev Cell* 2002;3:25-38.

[70] Yamauchi T, Kamon J, Minokoshi Y, Ito Y, Waki H, Uchida S, Yamashita S, Noda M, Kita S, Ueki K, Eto K, Akanuma Y, Froguel P, Foufelle F, Ferre P, Carling D, Kimura S, Nagai R, Kahn BB, Kadowaki T: Adiponectin stimulates glucose utilization and fatty-acid oxidation by activating AMP-activated protein kinase. *Nat Med* 2002;8:1288-1295.

[71] Bauchc IB, El Mkadem SA, Pottier A-M, Senou M, Many M-C, Rezsohazy R, Penicaud L, Maeda N, Funahashi T, Brichard SM: Overexpression of adiponectin targeted to adipose tissue in transgenic mice: impaired adipocyte differentiation. *Endocrinology* 2007;148:1539-1549.

[72] Eriksson P, Reynisdottir S, Lönnqvist F, Stemme V, Hamsten A, Arner P: Adipose tissue secretion of plasminogen activator inhibitor-1 in non-obese and obese individuals. *Diabetologia* 1998;41:65-71.

[73] Wolff SP, Dean RT: Glucose autoxidation and protein modification. The potential role of "autoxidative glycosylation" in diabetes. *Biochem* J 1987; 245:243-250.

[74] Brownlee M: Negative consequences of glycation. *Metab Clin Exp* 2000;49(Suppl 1):9-13.

[75] Requena JR, Fu MX, Ahmed MU, Jenkins AJ, Lyons TJ, Thorpe SR: Lipoxidation products as biomarkers of oxidative damage to proteins during lipid peroxidation reactions. *Nephrol Dial Transplant* 1996;11(Suppl 5):48-53.

[76] Busserolles J, Gueux E, Rock E, Mazur A, Rayssiguier Y: Substituting honey for refined carbohydrates protects rats from hypertriglyceridemic and prooxidative effects of fructose. *J Nutr* 2002;11:3379-3382.

[77] Faure P, Rossini E, Lafond JL, Richards MJ, Favier A, Halimi S: Vitamin E improves the free radical defense system potential and insulin sensitivity of rats fed high fructose diets. *J Nutr* 1997;127:103-107.

[78] MacDonald RB: Influence of dietary sucrose on biological aging. *Am J Clin Nutr* 1995;62:284S-293S.

[79] Busserolles J, Rock E, Gueux E, Mazur A, Grolier P, Rayssiguier Y: Short term consumption of a high sucrose diet has a pro-oxidant effect in rats. Br *J Nutr* 2002;87:337-342.

[80] Busserolles J, Zimowska W, Rock E, Raissiguier Y, Mazur A: Rats fed a high sucrose diet have altered heart antioxidant enzyme activity and gene expression. *Life Sci* 2002;71:1303-1312.

[81] Nandhini ATA, Thirunavukkarasu V, Ravichandran MK, Anuradha CV: Effect of taurine on biomarkers of oxidative stress in tissues of fructose-fed insulin-resistant rats. *Singapore Med J* 2005;46:82-87.

[82] Thirunavukkarasu V, Anitha Nandhini AT, Anuradha CV: Cardiac lipids and antioxidant status in high fructose rats and the effect of alpha-lipoic acid. *Nutr Metab Cardiovasc Dis* 2004;14:351-357.

[83] Wheeler MD, Nakagami M, Bradford BU, Uesugi T, Mason RP, Connor HD, Dikalova A, Kadiiska M, Thurman RG: Overexpression of manganese superoxide dismutase prevents alcohol-induced liver injury in the rat. *J Biol Chem* 2001;276:36664-36672.

[84] Dringen R: Metabolism and functions of glutathione in brain. *Progress Neurobiol* 2000;62:649-671.

[85] Pincemail J, Bonjean K, Cayeux K, Defraigne JO: Physiological action of antioxidant defenses. *Nutrition Clinique et Métabolisme* 2002;16:233-239.

[86] Girard A, Madani S, El Boustani ES, Belleville J, Prost J: Changes in lipid metabolism and antioxidant defense status in spontaneously hypertensive rats and Wistar rats fed a diet enriched with fructose and saturated fatty acids. *Nutrition* 2005;21:240-248.

[87] Martín-Gallán P, Carrascosa A, Gussinyé M, Domínguez C: Biomarkers of diabetes-associated oxidative stress and antioxidant status in young diabetic patients with or without subclinical complications. *Free Radic Biol Med* 2003;34:1563-1574.

[88] Atli T, Keven K, Avci A, Kutlay S, Turkcapar N, Varli M, Aras S, Ertug E, Canbolat O: Oxidative stress and antioxidant status in elderly diabetes mellitus and glucose intolerance patients. *Arch Gerontol Geriatr* 2004;39:269-275.

[89] Efe H, Rirci D, Deber O, Yildirmis S, Uydu HA, Orem C: Erytrhocyte antioxidant enzyme activities and lipid peroxidation in patients with types IIb and IV hyperlipoproteinemias. *Tohoku J Exp Med* 2004;202:163-172.

[90] Schettler V, Krontal J, Scheel A, Wieland E: No acute impact of lipid apheresis treatment on free radical scavenging enzyme gene expression in white blood cells. *Eur J Clin Invest* 2003;33:134-140.

[91] Montanaro A, Lombardo YB, González MS, Bernasconi AM, Chicco A, Rimoldi OJ, Bajabe JC, Brenner RR: Effect of troglitazone on the desaturases in a rat model of insulin-resistance induced by a sucrose-rich diet. *Prostaglandins Leukot Essent Fatty Acids* 2005;72:241-250.

[92] Reddy JK, Rao MS: Lipid metabolism and liver inflammation. II. Fatty liver disease and fatty acid oxidation. *Am J Physiol Gastrointest Liver Physiol* 2006;290:G852-G858.

[93] Ackerman Z, Oron-Herman M, Grozovski M, Rosenthal T, Pappo O, Link G, Sela BA: Fructose-induced fatty liver disease: hepatic effects of blood pressure and plasma triglyceride reduction. *Hypertension* 2005;45:1012-1018.

[94] Vrána A, Fábry P, Slabochová Z, Kazdová L: Effect of dietary fructose on free fatty acid release from adipose tissue and serum free fatty acid concentration in the rat. *Nutr Metab* 1974;17:74-83.

[95] Kamari Y, Grossman E, Oron-Herman M, Peleg E, Shabtay Z, Shamiss A, Sharabi Y: Metabolic stress with high carbohydrate diet increases adiponectin levels. *Horm Metab Res* 2007;39:384-388.

[96] Robertson PR: Chronic oxidative stress as a central mechanism for glucose toxicity in pancreatic islet beta cells in diabetes. *J Biol Chem* 2004;279:42351-42354.

[97] Kharroubi I, Ladriere L, Cardozo AK, Dogusan Z, Cnop M, Eizirik DL: Free fatty acids and cytokines induce pancreatic beta-cell apoptosis by different mechanisms: role of nuclear factor-kappa B and endoplasmic reticulum stress. *Endocrinology* 2004; 145:5087-5096.

[98] Del Zotto H, Borelli MI, Flores L, Garcia ME, Gomez Dumm CL, Chicco A, Lombardo YB, Gagliardino JJ: Islet neogenesis: an apparent key component of longterm pancreas adaptation to increased insulin demand. *J Endocrinol* 2004;183:321-330.

[99] Furukawa S, Fujita T, Shimabukuro M, Iwaki M, Yamada Y, Nakajima Y, Nakayama O, Makishima M, Matsuda M, Shimomura I: Increased oxidative stress in obesity and its impact on metabolic syndrome. *J Clin Invest* 2004;114:1752-1761.

[100] Brownlee M: The pathobiology of diabetic complications: a unifying mechanism. *Diabetes.* 2005;54:1615-1625.

In: Fructose
Editors: Brandon M. Johnston and Aaron B. Collins
ISBN: 978-1-62081-126-9

Chapter 2

HIGH-FRUCTOSE CONSUMPTION AND METABOLIC DISEASES

Cleide E. P. Trindade[1*], Cilmery Kurokawa[1], Rodrigo C. Barreiros[2], and Grasiela Bossolan[1]

[1]Department of Pediatrics, Botucatu School of Medicine, UNESP- São Paulo State University-Botucatu, São Paulo, Brazil

[2]Department of Medicine - Pediatrics
School of Medicine, Sorocaba, PUCSP-Sorocaba, São Paulo, Brazil

ABSTRACT

Renewed interest in the study of fructose arose after a number of papers on the harmful effects of ingesting high-fructose diets were published. Fructose intake has increased significantly in the United States and worldwide in the last four decades, which is mainly due to the increased consumption of high-fructose corn syrup and sucrose as a sweetener in beverages and in industrialized foods. There is substantial evidence from studies on rodents and on human adults suggesting that fructose intake in large amounts and for a long period of time leads to the development of the metabolic syndrome, insulin resistance, and dyslipidemia with increased plasma triacylglycerol, phospholipids and de novo lipogenesis. As a consequence, fructose may contribute to increased obesity, hypertension, type-2 diabetes and cardiovascular diseases. Fructose is a monosaccharide found in fruit, some vegetables and honey. Sucrose, a natural sweetener found in sugar cane and beets (50% fructose), is a disaccharide with two hexoses, one glucose molecule bonded to a fructose molecule by an alpha-1-4 glycoside. Although fructose has the same chemical formula as that of glucose ($C_6 H_{12} O_6$), it differs in its structure and metabolism. In the last few decades, sweeteners have been produced by corn starch hydrolysis, and part of the glucose produced is changed into fructose by enzymatic isomerization. This high-fructose corn syrup (42%-55% fructose) has a lower price than sucrose, and it has increasingly replaced sucrose as a sweetener in beverages and industrialized foods.

* Corresponding author: Department of Pediatrics, Division of Neonatology, Botucatu School of Medicine-UNESP-São Paulo State University, Rubião Júnior, CEP: 18618 970, Botucatu - São Paulo- Brazil, Tel.: +55 14 38116274; Fax: +55 14 38116274. E-mail address: cleidet@fmb.unesp.br

Fructose can be produced from glucose by the sorbitol pathway. In endogenous fructose production, non-phosphorylated glucose is converted into fructose. Initially, glucose produces sorbitol in a reaction catalyzed by aldose reductase. In the next step, fructose is formed from sorbitol in a reaction catalyzed by sorbitol dehydrogenase. This pathway may be important in the embryonic stages of human life for regeneration of pyridine nucleotides in order to maintain ATP concentrations and cellular redox potentials when the fetus is in a low oxygen environment. After absorption, fructose is rapidly extracted by the liver and metabolized into fructose-1-phosphate in a reaction catalyzed by fructokinase, which is specific for fructose. Subsequently, fructose-1-P is split by fructose-1-phosphate aldolase in trioses, dihydroxyacetone phosphate and glyceraldehyde, a pathway to provide the backbone for triacylglycerol and phospholipid synthesis. Triose-P is converted into glucose and glycogen as well as into lactate, which can produce plasma lactic acidosis, and into glycerol, a precursor for triglycerides and de novo lipogenesis. Although considerable evidence suggests that high fructose intake can produce harmful effects, investigations where high-fructose diets are compared with high-glucose diets are necessary to clarify the real role played by free fructose in adverse metabolic effects. In epidemiological studies, the analysis of the effects of high-fructose corn syrup and high sucrose intake must consider that both products are composed of fructose and glucose.

INTRODUCTION

Fructose is a carbohydrate found in plants and humans. It was isolated in 1947 from sugar cane, where it is a component of sucrose. The word fructose originates from the Latin *fructus* as fruits are an important source of fructose. Fructose is considered a sugar and the word sugar is derived from the Sanskrit *çarkara* which means grain of sand. From this Sanskrit word came the Greek word *sakkaron*, the Latin word *saccharum*, and the Arabic word *sukkar*.

Free fructose is normally ingested with diet, as a component of honey, fruits, and some vegetables. It is also synthesized in the organism from glucose through the sorbitol pathway. In normal cellular metabolism this pathway is related to oxy-reductive process and regeneration of pyridine nucleotides.

Interest in studying fructose was renewed after many papers appeared on the harmful effects of high fructose diets. There is substantial evidence from studies in human adults suggesting that high fructose diets can induce metabolic syndrome, insulin resistance, and increased de novo lipogenesis which results in increased plasma triacylglycerol, phosphorlipids and cholesterol. As a consequence high fructose diets may contribute to obesity, Type 2 diabetes, hyperuricemia, high blood pressure, and cardiovascular diseases.

Early studies focused on its role as a glucose substitute in medical practice. Some studies suggested that fructose may be beneficial to individuals who are overweight, have non-insulin dependent diabetes mellitus, or participate in exercise activities [1]. However the clinical benefits conflict with harmful effects like ATP consumption, hypertriglyceridemia, and lactacidemia. Presently, its use is limited to specific situations such as a sport drink during endurance exercises.

In the last few years, fructose consumption has significantly increased as many Industrialized products use high-fructose corn syrups in place of sucrose to sweeten processed foods and beverages like bakery products, juices, and candies.

This chapter will present an overview of the fructose metabolism, possible uses, and the harmful effects when it is consumed in high quantities over long periods.

Biochemical Characteristics

Fructose is a monosaccharide with six carbon atoms linked, by simple covalent bonds, to hydroxyl groups formed by hydrogen and oxygen, and a carbonyl group with a double bond, linking carbon to oxygen. The position of this group determines whether carbohydrate hydrolysis will result in a ketone or an aldehyde. As fructose has the carbonyl group -CO- at the end of the chain, when hydrolyzed it produces ketone. For this reason fructose is considered a ketohexose. Although fructose has the same chemical formula as glucose ($C_6 H_{12} O_6$) it differs in structure and metabolism. Glucose has the carbonyl group in the first carbon and when hydrolyzed produces aldehyde. Carbohydrate oxidation is the main pathway for producing energy in most cells.

Sources of Fructose

Fructose, also called levulose (D-fructose), can be found in fruits and honey as an isolated carbohydrate, or as a component in more complex carbohydrates like sucrose, and polymers like fructosan, e.g. inuline, found in certain tubers. Sucrose, a natural sweetener found in large quantities in sugar cane and beets (50% fructose), is a disaccharide with two hexoses, one molecule of glucose linked to one molecule of fructose by an alpha 1-4 glycosidic bond [2]. Raffinose, a trisaccharide found in cotton seed and sugar beet molasses, is composed of D-glucose, D-fructose, and D-galactose, and is formed by the transfer of galactose from UDP-galactose to sucrose.

Fructose can result from oxidation of sorbitol in a reaction mediated by sorbitol dehydrogenase. Sorbitol is present in many plants, particularly apple, pear, cherry, plum, and apricot. Table 1 shows the fructose, glucose, and sucrose content of several foods.

In the seventies, high performance liquid chromatography facilitated the separation of fructose from sugars. This method increased the production of a pure form of fructose and decreased its price. As well as isolating an isomerase which could transform D-glucose in D-fructose [4], contributed to the commercial introduction of high-fructose corn syrup (HFCS), a corn starch syrup rich in fructose. HFCS-42 (42% fructose) was introduced in 1967 and HFCS-55 (55% fructose) in 1977. HFCS-42 is 1.16 times and HFCS-55 1.28 times as sweet as sucrose [4]. This high-fructose corn syrup is cheaper than sucrose and has increasingly replaced sucrose as a sweetener in beverages and industrialized foods [6]. Fructose is highly soluble in water solutions and very sweet, 1.7 times the sweetness of sucrose, favoring its use over sucrose. Bakery foods contain between 1.0% and 2.05% fructose and if fruits are added this may increase to nearly 11.0%. Honey is high in fructose, 42.4%, and is considered a natural sweetener [6].

Table 1. Sugar contents of foods, g/100g

Foods	Fructose	Glucose	Sucrose
Apple	7.6	2.3	3.3
Apple juice	5.5	2.5	1.7
Apricot, raw	0.7	1.6	5.2
Apricot, dried	12.2	20.3	6.4
Bananas	2.7	4.2	6.5
Blackberries	4.1	3.1	0.4
Blueberries	3.6	3.5	0.2
Cherries	6.2	8.1	0.2
Figs, raw	2.8	3.7	0.4
Figs, dried	26.0	28.6	6.5
Grapes	6.9	6.6	1.4
Orange raw	2.5	2.2	4.2
Orange juice, raw	3.0	2.8	4.1
Pears raw	6.4	1.9	1.8
Pear juice, raw	7.1	1.6	-
Honey	41	34	2
Asparagus	1.3	0.9	0.2
Beets	0.2	0.2	6.1
Broccoli	0.7	0.6	0.3
Carrots	1.0	1.0	3.6
Cauliflower	0.8	0.9	0.5
Tomato	1.4	1.1	0.0

Adapted from Mathews et al. (1987), ref. [3], and Hallffrisch (1990), ref. [14].

FRUCTOSE CONSUMPTION

Carbohydrate intake in the Western World is 200-300g/day corresponding to between 40% and 50% of ingested energy. In the United States, mean daily fructose intake is 16g/day and 31g/day at the 90 percentile; if corn syrup is added this may reach 60-100g/day, or even 150g/day if sucrose is added [7].

Added sweeteners are important components of the American diet and from 1994 to 1996, represented 318kcal of dietary intake and 16% of total caloric intake. There is no doubt that fructose ingestion has increased in the last few decades in the United States, the highest consumers being teenagers and young adults, and sweet beverages the most important source of fructose intake [2].

In 1970, reports from the United States Department of Agriculture (USDA) indicated that the per capita added sugar in the American diet was 90/g day and no HFCS was consumed. Between 1970 and 1985 HFCS consumption increased and sucrose intake decreased [2]. USDA dietary records from 1977-1978 indicated mean daily fructose intake was 37g in the United States population [8]. In this survey sugar sweetened-beverages appeared as the mainly source of fructose in all age classes. The exception was for children under 6 years and adults over 50 years [8]. In an interesting review article, Tappy and Lê [2] analyzed the evolution of fructose intake. The authors found that from 1977 to 1990 average daily fructose intake was 54.7g, corresponding to an increase of 46% in a 10 to 16 year period (The Third National Health and Nutrition Examination Survey-NHANES III). Assessment of the evolution of fructose intake from 1999 to 2004 indicated that average fructose consumption was 49g/day and accounted for 42% of all calories from sweeteners consumed (NHANES 1999-2004) [2].

Although the United States is the main HFCS user in the world, HFCS is now produced and used in other countries, but data is scant. South America and Oceania are the highest sugar consumers; the lowest are Asia and Africa [2].

In Brazil, a sugar exporting country, mean fructose ingestion from fruit and vegetables is 4.34g/day, and from sucrose, 27.5g/day. This estimate was based on statistical data of alimentary ingested products, from the 1995/6 survey of Brazilian family budgets (IBGE-8) [9].

METABOLIC ASPECTS OF FRUCTOSE

Intestinal absorption

Fructose absorption across the small intestine is performed by two different mechanisms. Absorption takes place via a facilitated transport, independent from glucose, with a slower absorption rate than glucose and galactose, and by a glucose-dependent high capacity co-transport [10].

Fructose, present at the brush-border membrane, is transported into the enterocyte through a specific fructose transporter, GLUT5, located at the apical pole of the enterocyte. This transporter has a high affinity for fructose and low affinity for glucose. Fructose is transported throughout the enterocyte by the GLUT2 transporter, situated at the basolateral pole of the enterocyte.

The capacity of human adults to absorb fructose is limited and symptoms of malabsorption such as diarrhea and flatulence have been reported after fructose loading. This effect is largely abolished when fructose is ingested with glucose possibly due to activation of the fructose transporter by glucose [1, 11]. Fructose absorption is increased when ingested as sucrose or ingested with glucose. During glucose absorption small solutes, including fructose, move passively through opened junctions increasing fructose absorption by 29% [12]. Malabsorption rates for fructose and sorbitol are very similar in all studies. They vary according to the quantity and concentration of the sugar. After a 50g load of fructose in a 20% solution, 60% to 70% of patients display malabsorption [13].

Hepatic Metabolism

First Steps of Fructose and Glucose Metabolism

Fructose is mainly metabolized in the liver, although the intestines and kidneys have the enzymes necessary for its metabolism. A small proportion of orally administered fructose may be converted to glucose and lactate during transport through the intestinal wall [2].

After absorption, the fructose present in portal blood is rapidly extracted by hepatocytes. Although fructose is absorbed more slowly than glucose, it is more rapidly metabolized by the liver. The rapid fructose entrance into liver cells is mediated by the GLUT2 transporter. This process takes place without energy expenditure or insulin stimulation. Differently to glucose, fructose only has a modest effect on the stimulation of insulin secretion and does not require the presence of insulin to enter the intracellular compartment [1].

The initial steps of hepatic glucose metabolism differ from those of fructose, where different enzymes and reactions take place. Glucose is converted into glucose-6-P under hexokinase or glucokinase enzyme action. Glucose-6-P is converted to fructose-6-P and to fructose-1,6-di-P through a reaction catalyzed by the enzyme phosphofructokinase. Subsequently fructose-1,6-di-P is cleaved into two trioses, di-hydroxyacetone-P and glyceraldehyde-3-P (Figure 1). The metabolites from fructose-1,6-di-P will further be converted into pyruvate that enters the Krebs cycle to produce ATP and CO_2. The conversion of glucose to pyruvate is regulated by the energy status of cells, and by insulin that stimulates glucokinase gene expression and the activation of glycolytic enzymes [2].

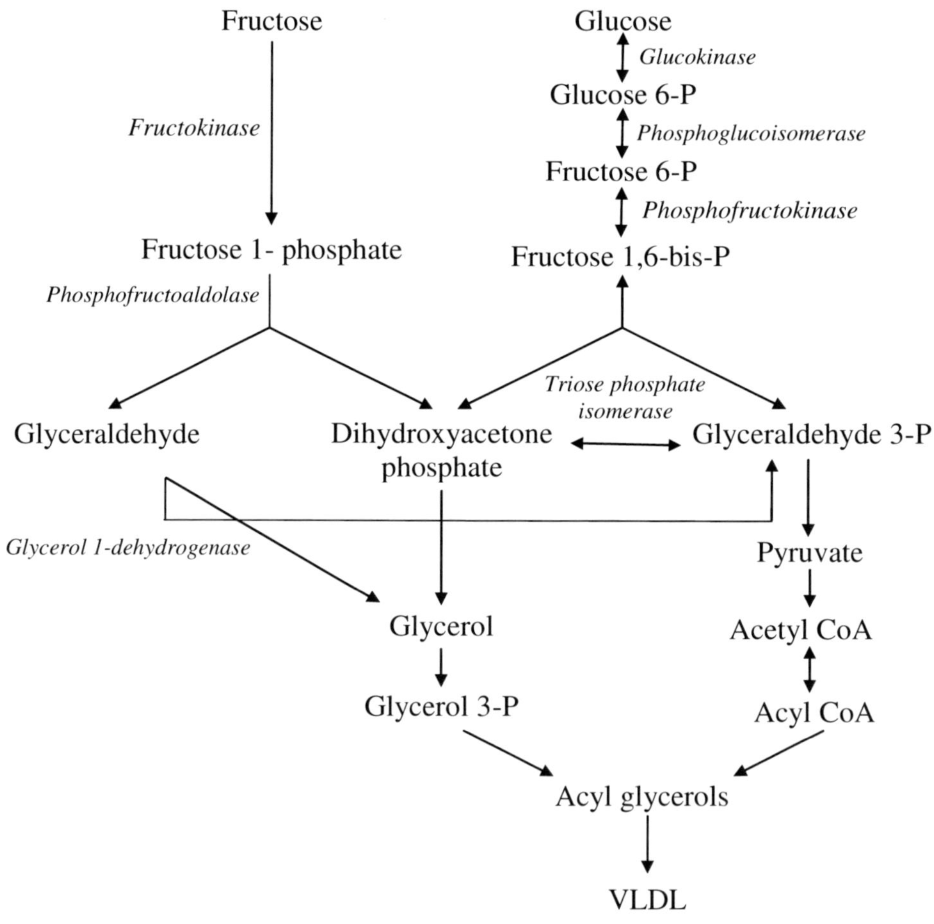

Figure 1. Fructose and glucose metabolism. Possible fructose metabolic pathway to generate triacylglycerol synthesis.

A large part of fructose uptake from the portal vein occurs immediately during the first pass in the liver. Once inside the cell, fructose is rapidly phosphorylated on carbon one in a reaction mediated by fructokinase, a fructose specific enzyme, and is converted to fructose-1-phosphate. This phosphorylation bypasses the initial limiting steps of insulin-stimulated transport needed for glucose metabolism. The increase in fructose intake stimulates increased fructokinase activity [14]. Further, fructose-1-phosphate is cleaved by aldolase B into two trioses: di-hydroxyacetone phosphate and glyceraldehyde, rather than glyceraldehyde-3-P which is directly produced in glucose metabolism. Di-hydroxiacetone phosphate can be isomerized into glyceraldehyde-3-phosphate. Glyceraldehyde from fructose is further phosphorylated to glyceraldehyde-3-P. This is the point where fructose metabolism is interrelated with glucose metabolism.

Metabolic Fate of Triose-P from Fructose

Triose-P derived from fructose can be further metabolized in different ways. The major part of triose-P is converted to glucose and glycogen through gluconeogenesis [2,15] (Figure 1). About two thirds of fructose is converted to glucose, which may accumulate as glycogen, be released from liver as glucose [1], or be oxidized in extrahepatic tissues [2].

Triose-P may be metabolized in the glycolytic pathway and then converted into lactate and pyruvate. A significant increase in plasma lactate can be observed after oral or intravenous fructose intake, and has been associated with lactic acidosis. Under normal circumstances, small amounts of fructose can be converted into pyruvate and oxidized to carbon dioxide through the tricarboxylic acid cycle. Before pyruvate entrance in the citric acid cycle it must be oxidatively decarboxylated to acetyl-Co-A, the source of carbon for fatty acid synthesis. Only a small proportion of fructose is converted to de novo fatty acids (Figure 1) [16].

Part of the glyceraldehyde produced is phosphorylated by a specific kinase to glyceroldehyde-3-P, a precursor of glucose production through gluconeogenesis. Part is reduced to glycerol by the action of glycerol 1-dehydrogenase and then phosphorylated to provide glycerol-3-P, a precursor in the synthesis of acylglycerols and other lipid products by de novo lipogenesis [14,17] (Figure 1).

The bulk of blood triacyglycerol is carried in 2 lipoprotein particles: chylomicrons and VLDL particles. Chylomicrons are produced by the intestine and are found in low concentrations in blood during fasting. These particles contain proteins, apolipoprotein B-48, and carry triacylglycerol derived from ingested fat. VLDL particles are produced by the liver, contain apolipoprotein B-100, and carry endogenous triacylglycerol. Concentrations of apo B-48, the apolipoprotein from chylomicrons, are normally 6 times lower (0.01μmol/L or 0.3mg/dL) than those of VLDL apo B-100 (0.06μmol/L or 3mg/dL) in the fasting state. Blood triacylglycerol (20% to 50%) can be carried in remnants of VLDL called intermediate-density lipoproteins (IDLs) [18].

The adverse effects of high fructose intake are related to the amount of fructose and the length of time that a person remains on a high fructose diet. Rats fed a high fructose diet, exhibit characteristics of metabolic syndrome which include insulin resistance, hyperinsulinemia, hypertriglyceridemia, and hypertension. The adverse effects were related to the amount and duration of fructose consumption [19]. There is evidence from studies of at least 4 weeks dietary control that diets containing ≥20% energy as fructose can cause lipid abnormalities like hypertriglyceridemia due to VLDL-triglyceride increases when associated with hyperinsulinemia, and LDL-cholesterol increases in normoinsulinemic subjects [20]. A discretely lower amount of fructose, >15% of energy as fructose, was associated with increases in both fasting and postprandial triacylglycerol in humans [16]. In perfused liver, fructose inhibited hepatic lipid oxidation and facilitated fatty acid reesterification and VLDL-triglyceride synthesis [21].

As fructose can be metabolized by different pathways, more studies are needed to identify the contribution, and possible effects on human health, of each metabolic pathway. In a study investigating the effects of fructose or glucose meals on postprandial lipemia in 14 healthy subjects, the authors used stable isotopes, [$2H_2$]palmitate and [$U^{13}C$]D-fructose or [$U^{13}C$]D-glucose to trace the fate of dietary sugars [16]. Post-meal plasma triacylglycerol concentration was higher and rose earlier after fructose than glucose ingestion. The authors concluded that the contribution of de novo fatty acids to the increase of VLDL-triglycerides (VLDL-TG) by fructose is small. In contrast, de novo TG-glycerol formed from labeled fructose made up 38% of circulating VLDL-TG 240 minutes after fructose ingestion. Only 35% of the fructose load was oxidized over 6 hours. Approximately 40% of the remaining fructose was transformed into lactate and glycogen. The authors concluded that fructose contribution to de novo triacylglycerol synthesis through glycerol production is more significant than its contribution through fatty acid production. The conclusion was that a decrease in plasma-TG removal, via a lower activation of adipose tissue lipoprotein lipase, contributes to acute fructose-induced lipemia [16,18,20]. The exact contribution from lipoprotein lipase needs to be clarified. Not only in humans was decreased triglyceride clearance considered a contributory factor to high triacylglycerol levels, but studies using rats fed high-fructose diets also lead to the conclusion that both fructose and sucrose increased triglyceride production and decreased triglyceride clearance [16,22].

Endogenous Fructose Production

An interesting aspect of fructose metabolism is endogenous fructose production by the sorbitol pathway. Sorbitol is frequently ingested with food as it is found mainly in fruits, or can be produced from glucose as an alternative pathway in glucose metabolism (Figure 2). In this pathway, fructose is created in the liver directly from glucose supplied by the blood through the intermediate formation of its corresponding alcohol, D-sorbitol. This pathway has not been fully studied in humans and its real function and contribution to the total fructose pool is unknown.

It is has long been known that human spermatozoa live in a fructose environment produced by the prostate gland and seminal vesicles. The metabolic pathway includes aldose reductase and sorbitol dehydrogenase. The same process may occur in the liver, nerve tissue, and muscle [23]. The polyol pathway has also been identified in plants and animal tissues [24].

Ungulate animal placentas produce fructose and high fructose concentrations are found in fetal blood. Biochemical evidence has shown that fetal fructose in these animals is produced in the placenta from maternal glucose [25,26]. In the human fetus and newborn, data on polyols and sugars other than glucose, are scarce and their roles in placental, fetal, and postnatal metabolism need to be defined [27], Fructose, sorbitol, inositol, erythritol, and ribitol in coelomic and amniotic fluid from 5 to 12 week gestation embryos [28], and sorbitol in cord blood from full-term newborns have been found at higher levels than maternal concentrations, suggesting that the polyol pathway is active in the fetus [29].

In endogenous fructose production, non-phosphorylated glucose is converted into fructose (Figure 2). In a first step, glucose, in a reaction catalyzed by aldose reductase, generates sorbitol and NADPH is oxidized to $NADP^+$. In the second step, fructose is formed from sorbitol in a reaction catalyzed by sorbitol dehydrogenase and NAD^+ is reduced to NADH, a co-factor that under anaerobic conditions is reoxidized by the conversion of pyruvate to lactate which can result in increased blood lactate [1,28,30]. NAD^+ allows the glycolisis process to continue and produce ATP [14,28,31]. This route bypasses the ordinary glucose metabolism pathways, in which phosphorylated derivatives are intermediates.

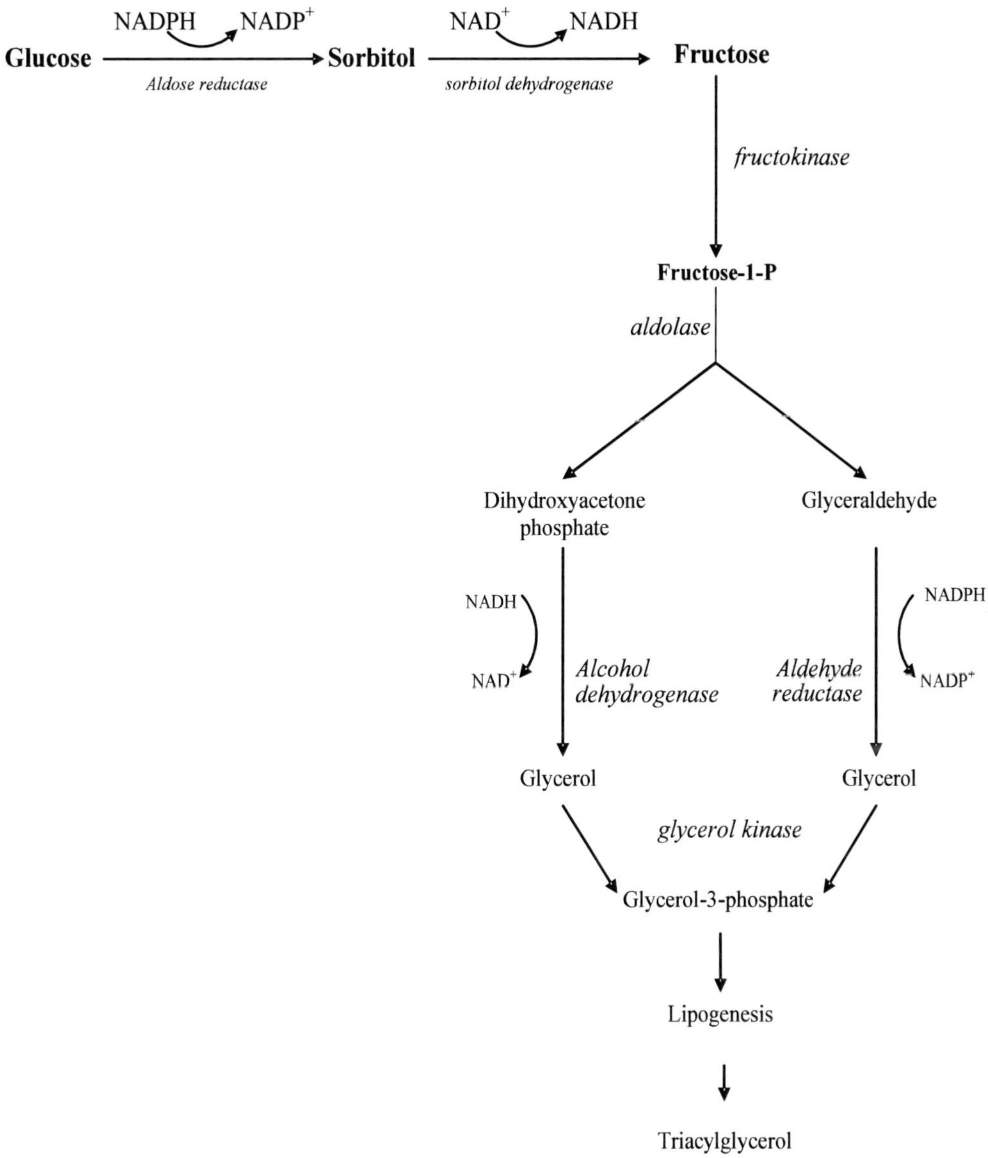

Figure 2. Schematic representation of fructose production and metabolism via the polyol pathway.

Many papers have been published concerning the harmful effects of high–fructose diets on human adults. In contrast few papers refer to obese children and high fructose diet [32], and one investigated fructose in coelomic and amniotic fluid from 5-12 week gestation embryos showing the presence of fructose in early life [28]. The lack of studies in this vulnerable period of life stimulated us to investigate fructose in fetus (cord blood) and the newborn infant to identify its presence in the early perinatal period and to find a physiological role for it.

In our study [33], investigating the presence of fructose in maternal blood and umbilical cord blood, and in peripheral blood from the normal full-term newborn 48h after delivery, we could observe that fructose concentrations in fetal blood were significantly higher than in maternal blood, suggesting endogenous fructose production by the fetus via the sorbitol pathway. The highest fructose values were found in newborns 48h after birth suggesting that fructose production is a continuous process from fetus to newborn infant. Considering that the newborns were breast-fed and that analysis of their breast milk showed it did not contain sorbitol or fructose, we concluded that fructose originated from glucose or glycogen through the sorbitol pathway [33]. From the beginning we had two questions: why the fetus uses an alternative pathway to the glucose metabolism to produce fructose, considering that glucose is a very important carbohydrate in producing energy for fetal and newborn brain and growth. The second was about the destiny of the endogenous fructose produced.

Besides a suggestion in literature [28] that fructose pathways play a role in reoxidation of pyridine nucleotides during the early stages of gestation, we hypothesized that fructose may be a precursor for lipid synthesis in the fetus and newborn. This hypothesis is based on the concept that fructose is more lipogenic than glucose and from analyzing the lipogenic effects of high-fructose diets in humans. At 50% to 60% gestation there is little lipid uptake by the fetus, mainly the essential fatty acids necessary for membrane development. In the last trimester of gestation large amounts of body fat are deposited (12% to 18% of body weight). The importance of this adiposity and the mechanisms that produce it are not well known. Considering that neutral lipids do not pass through the placental barrier, they must be produced by the fetus, thus fructose may contribute to the carbon backbone for triacylglycerol production in the fetus, and also in the newborn as seen in sheep fetuses [34]. In that article the [^{14}C] derived from [^{14}C] glucose and [^{14}C] fructose infused in fetal circulation was incorporated into neutral lipids and phospholipids from the heart, liver, kidney, brain, and adipose tissue. The incorporation patterns from fructose and glucose were similar.

Ectopic Lipid Deposition

Literature is scarce on intrahepatocellular (IHCL) and intramyocellular (IMCL) accumulation of lipids as a consequence of high-fructose diets in humans. Triglyceride deposition in hepatocyte cytoplasm leads to nonalcoholic liver disease. In rodents, a high-fructose diet induces hepatic insulin resistance, IHCL, and stimulates hepatic de novo lipogenesis [35]. High-fructose or sucrose ingested for long periods may induce hepatic steatosis, insulin resistance, and IMCL accumulation [36,37,38]. In healthy subjects with and without a family history of Type 2 diabetes submitted to a 7-day isocaloric diet or hypercaloric high-fructose diet, the authors concluded that the high-fructose diet increased fasting VLDL-triacylglycerol, induced ectopic lipid deposition in liver and muscle, and decreased hepatic insulin sensitivity. The high-fructose diet increased VLDL-triacylglycerols and IMCL to a greater extent in healthy offspring of subjects with a family history of Type 2 diabetes. This group appeared more susceptible to the adverse effects of high-fructose diets [37]. These characteristics were considered indicators of genetically determined metabolic alterations [37].

Fructose and Exercise

During prolonged exercise blood glucose levels fall and muscle glycogen depletion occurs. This limits athletic performance. Ingestion of carbohydrate solution, prior to 60 minutes or longer of high-intensity exercise can delay fatigue and improve endurance performance, by preventing hypoglycemia and by maintaining a high carbohydrate-oxidation rate. This is important during the later stage of exercise, when endogenous muscle and liver carbohydrate stores may be depleted [1]. The contribution by exogenous glucose to energy provision during prolonged high-intensity endurance exercise is limited to ~1.0-1.1g/min, even when ingested in quantities that exceed this rate. This could be explained by saturation of sodium-dependent glucose co-transporter (SGLT1) which is located in the brush-border membrane of the small intestine and is responsible for absorption of glucose by active transport [39].

Literature shows that glucose intake during endurance exercises has beneficial effects. However, glucose stimulates insulin and suppresses glucagon secretion. Fructose, on the contrary, produces minimal changes in blood glucose, insulin, and glucagon levels and is considered a more ideal energy source during prolonged exercises [1]. Although fructose has some advantages over glucose as an energy source, there are conflicting reports in literature, and it has been suggested that fructose, as a supplement in sports drinks, may have little advantage over glucose ingestion during endurance exercise [1].

There are benefits in the association of glucose and fructose. During exercise, fructose ingested with glucose increases exogenous carbohydrate oxidation rate up to 1.75g/min compared with 1g/min during exercise with glucose alone [40,41]. Fructose ingested with glucose increased intestinal glucose transport. This could explain the increase in glucose oxidation rate [40-42].

Plasma lactate increases during exercise when fructose and glucose are ingested together compared to isoenergetic amounts of glucose or glucose polymers. This could have a beneficial effect because lactate is efficiently oxidized by active muscles during exercise [43,44]. In a study with human volunteers, LeCoutre et al. observed that co-ingestion of fructose and glucose prior to exercise lead to an increase in carbohydrate oxidation rate, due essentially to enhanced lactate oxidation [45].

Effects of Dietary Fructose

Dyslipidemia

Although many publications in literature address the effects of dietary fructose on lipid metabolism in humans, analyses must take into account that in high-fructose diets, fructose is ingested together with glucose as a component of sucrose, or as HFCS which is composed of fructose and glucose. Administration of equivalent quantities of pure fructose, sucrose, a mixture of glucose and fructose, or HFCS resulted in similar postprandial increases in triglycerides [46]. Also many of the health problems induced by fructose are similar to diseases produced by overeating, high-fat diets, and high-carbohydrate diets. High-fructose/high-sucrose diets lead to adverse metabolic effects and cause dyslipidemia, insulin resistance, hypertension, hyperuricemia, and obesity [2]. Although animal studies have been described since 1970 [47,48], the bulk of literature on dietary fructose and human health has only appeared in the last twenty years.

Some human groups are more susceptible to presenting hypertriglyceridemia from fructose intake; these include the male gender, post menopause women, hyperinsulinemic men, previous hypertriglyceridemia, and Type 2 diabetes [14].

In 2000, Bantle et al. [49] reported gender differences when feeding men and women for 6 weeks on a diet providing 17% of energy as fructose, and a diet sweetened with glucose. In men, the fructose diet significantly increased fasting, postprandial, and daylong plasma triacylglycerol concentrations compared to the glucose diet. In women, fructose had no effect. The reason for this gender difference was not clear. Also, triacylglycerol concentrations were higher in men than women after 24h ingestion of HFCS or sucrose sweetened beverages [46]. These data suggest that men are more susceptible than women to the effects of sugars containing fructose [46].

In an investigation of the mechanisms of the acute effect of fructose on postprandial lipemia, the authors used stable isotopes to trace the metabolism and the fate of dietary fructose and glucose [16]. Plasma triacylglycerol and VLDL-triacylglycerol concentrations were higher whereas the concentration of insulin and $[^2H_2]$palmitate in nonesterified fatty acids were lower after fructose than after glucose diets. The conclusion was that the lower insulin secretion after fructose ingestion may result in less activation of adipose lipoprotein lipase and impairment of triacylglycerol clearance. Therefore, two mechanisms seem to be responsible for the increased triacylglycerol, de novo lipogenesis, and decreased triacylglycerol clearance. Also de novo lipogenesis from fructose contributes to the partitioning of fatty acids toward esterification [16].

A systematic review and meta-analysis assembled sixteen clinical trials and included 236 subjects to compare the effects of isocaloric fructose and carbohydrates. The following lipids were analyzed in Type 1 and Type 2 diabetic subjects: triglycerides, total cholesterol, LDL cholesterol, and HDL cholesterol. Increasing triglyceride and lowering total cholesterol was observed only in subjects with Type 2 diabetes when starch was the reference carbohydrate. These effects were not observed when fructose was compared to sucrose or mixed carbohydrate as reference because both sources contained fructose [50].

Fructose at >60g/day used as a sweetener raised triglycerides in ≥4 weeks follow-up [50]. Young adults and women who consumed glucose, fructose, and HFCS-sweetened beverages at 25% of energy requirements for 2 weeks, had the 24h triglyceride area under the curve increased during consumption of fructose compared with baseline, and fasting low-density lipoprotein (LDL) and apoB concentrations increased during ingestion of fructose and HFCS [51]. These authors estimated that 13% of the United States population consumes 25% or more of its energy from added sugar, and therefore this population are at risk of cardiovascular diseases [51].

A meta-analysis which evaluated the effects of dietary fructose concluded that an intake >50g/day was associated with increased postprandial triglyceride excursions, whereas a fructose intake >100g/day was associated with increased fasting triglycerides [2,52]. The estimates of fructose intake, based on NHANES 1999-2004, revealed that young men in the 15-18 and 19-22 years age groups had the highest estimated mean intake of total fructose, 75g/day. Women had lower estimated fructose intakes than men in all age groups, 48.6g/day versus 62.8g/day. Total estimated mean usual daily fructose intake in both genders and all ages was 49g/day, very close to the amount considered a risk factor for increased postprandial triglyceride excursions [53].

Obesity and Fructose

The increase in obesity worldwide over the last decade has been considered an important public health matter, principally because obesity is associated to comorbidities like: metabolic syndrome, insulin resistance, Type 2 diabetes, hypertension, and coronary artery disease. The concomitant increase in soft drink consumption, sweetened with sucrose or HFCS, suggests a relationship between fructose and the obesity epidemic [2,5,54,55], especially in young people and children [56,57].

Epidemiological studies support the association between high sugar intake, adiposity, and body weight increase. Some reports are descriptive and results contradictory. Although there is no doubt that fructose may produce acute and long term increases in blood triglycerides and visceral lipids it is important to recognize that fat diets, sedentary lifestyle, socioeconomic factors, hormones, and genetics are also contributive factors to obesity. Obesity is a very complex state which involves the regulation of food intake, energy expenditure, and body fat stores by different nutrients, hormones, and the central nervous system [48]. Endocrine regulators of energy homeostasis, like leptin, insulin, ghrelin, and possibly peptide YY_{3-36} from the distal intestine, are released in proportion to body fat, to the quantity and composition of food consumed [48]. Some experiments support a relationship between fructose and the behavior of hormones that regulate energy homeostasis.

To understand the real effect of fructose on human health it is important to analyze studies in which free fructose is compared to glucose, even though these diets are not used in daily life, but only in experiments. Experimental studies in mice with free access to fructose (15% solution in water), sucrose 10%, or artificial sweetener (0% of calories), showed that animals in the fructose group had greater increases in body weight and body fat than the animals in the sucrose and artificial sweetener groups. Also, fructose supplementation impaired glucose tolerance, but had no influence on insulin, adiponectin, and ghrelin levels [58]. In human subjects the consumption of fructose-sweetened beverages compared to glucose-sweetened beverages reduced insulin secretion, leptin production, and attenuated ghrelin suppression [59]. Consumption of fructose or glucose-sweetened beverages at 25% of energy requirements demonstrated that fructose increased visceral adipose deposition and de novo lipogenesis, but decreased glucose tolerance, insulin sensitivity in older, overweight and obese men and woman [60]. These effects were not observed with glucose ingestion.

Insulin plays a role in regulating body adiposity by its action in the central nervous system which leads to inhibition of food intake, and increased energy expenditure [48]. Insulin receptors are expressed in several CNS areas related to the control of food intake and energy homeostasis [61]. Fructose is a weak stimulator of insulin secretion probably because of the low expression level of fructose transporter GLUT5 in pancreatic β-cell. Leptin is produced by adipocytes and acts as a signal to the CNS in the regulation of food intake, energy expenditure, and body adiposity [62]. Together with insulin it acts in the hypothalamus and regulates food intake and energy metabolism via neuropeptide systems [51]. The leptin area under the curve over 24 hours was reduced by 20%-30% when normal weight women [59], and overweight men and women [63] consumed meals with fructose compared with glucose-sweetened beverages. In these studies, the presence of insulin resistance led to hypertriglyceridemia in response to glucose and fructose, but the intensity of the changes were higher with fructose.

Ghrelin is a peptide hormone produced by the stomach and upper small intestine. Its action is associated with food intake regulation [51]. Circulating ghrelin levels are inversely related to body weight and ghrelin increases after the intake of weight loss diets. Plasma ghrelin was 35% lower after meals accompanied by a glucose-sweetened beverage; but the decrease was greater after fructose-sweetened beverages [59].

Uric acid and Fructose

Increased dietary fructose intake has boosted research in various scientific fields. Studies on renal diseases and metabolic syndrome have linked increased fructose intake with high uric acid levels [64]. Fructose and its association with uric acid have been found in other disease situations; these include obesity/metabolic syndrome, gout, hypertension, diabetes, and heart and kidney diseases [2,65].

Uric acid seems to be an indicator of the toxic effect from high fructose intake [66], and its early formation, seen 30 minutes after ingesting the carbohydrate, reinforces the connection between fructose metabolism and uric acid formation. The action of hepatic fructokinase on that carbohydrate results in fructose 1-P, ADP, AMP, and uric acid [2]. Regulation of this pathway does not seem to suffer from the action of negative regulators, as observed in the glucose pathway, suggesting that excessive fructose intake, without proper control, can result in high uric acid levels.

Nakagawa et al (2005) observed that uric acid plays a fundamental role in the development of experimental metabolic syndrome. Treating these rats with allopurinol, a xanthine oxidase inhibitor which lowers uric acid levels, was able to decrease systolic blood pressure, increase insulin sensitivity and normalize triglyceride levels after the development of fructose-induced metabolic syndrome [67].

The capacity to produce uric acid from consuming large quantities of fructose seems to be influenced by genetic factors. Genetic polymorphism of the genes responsible for the synthesis of anion transporters such as Uric Acid Anion Transporter 1 (URAT-1) is associated with hyperuricemia [68]. Similarly to other enzymes or metabolic pathways, uric acid production also seems to be influenced by an individual's genetics and to be controlled by various genes and pathways [69]. Some individuals may produce high concentrations of uric acid whereas others may produce lower levels, suggesting a higher or lower susceptibility in certain individuals to the propensity and/or development of fructose-induced metabolic syndrome. Other studies have suggested that fructose may be produced by an individual's organism, and they report that this pathway may be an alternative pathway that complements the toxic effect of fructose and metabolic syndrome. Individuals with diabetes and severe insulin resistance seem to synthetize fructose from glucose by using the polyol pathway [33]. Another negative effect of induced uric acid production in this situation is the inhibition of endothelial NO synthesis, which has been observed in cell cultures and experimental models [67,70]. The capacity of uric acid from the fructose metabolism to inhibit NO (endogenous vasodilator) has been associated with hypertension and heart disease. Uric acid also has a direct toxic effect on adipocytes, causing inflammation and inducing oxidative stress. These findings on the role of uric acid seem controversial, considering that the uric acid is one of the main antioxidants in the circulation. Finally, further studies on the fructose metabolism and the role played by uric acid in microenvironments and specifics diseases are still needed. Clarifying the actual role played by uric acid in various diseases, its relationship with high fructose intake, its production, and inhibition pathways is still a challenge to be overcome.

Hypertension and Fructose

Animal studies have shown a clear association between fructose ingestion and hypertension [71]. Experimental studies in dogs fed the same levels of high fructose and glucose diets, showed a net difference in metabolic response, with high fructose leading to hypertension and other adverse effects [72]. An association was also seen in rats between high-fructose ingestion and the development of cardiac hypertrophy [73], reduced baroreflex sensitivity [74], and renal damage [75]. Ingestion of acute quantities of fructose in humans elicits an increase in blood pressure which is probably mediated by increased cardiac output without compensatory peripheral vasodilation. The contrast between fructose ingestion response and the same amount of glucose may be explained by insulin hemodynamic action, as fructose has a negligible effect on insulin secretion. Physiological elevations in plasma insulin concentrations produce a rise in cardiac output and a reduction in muscle and systemic vascular resistance [76].

The association between fructose and hypertension may be explained by the uric acid pathway. Excessive fructose consumption leads to increased serum uric acid via fructose phosphorylation, and the generation of adenosine diphosphate which is metabolized to uric acid. Increased uric acid levels are associated to reduced nitric oxide levels and thus to blood hypertension. Sugar consumption is also associated to enhanced sympathetic nervous system activity, and sodium retention [77].

Frutose is the only sugar that raises uric acid concentration because fructose enters into hepatocytes and other cells, including tubular cells, adipocytes, and intestinal epithelial cells, where it is completely metabolized by frutokinase. In this process ATP is consumed without a negative regulatory mechanism to prevent ATP depletion. This leads to increases in lactic acid and uric acid levels which can increase 1-4mg/dL after a large ingestion of fructose [78]. Uric acid is associated with hypertension and a large number of deleterious effects, mainly by the stimulation of vascular smooth muscle cell proliferation and release of chemotactic and inflammatory substances [79,80]. The mechanism by which uric acid causes hypertension may involve a reduction in the concentration of endothelial nitric oxide, which results in systemic and intrarenal vasoconstriction, renal microvascular disease, and systemic hypertension [78,81].

Other experiments give support to the hypothesis that fructose plays a role in the pathophysiology of hypertension. Studies with mice have shown that diets rich in fructose stimulated salt absorption in the small intestine and kidney tubules, and resulted a state of salt overload which caused hypertension [82]. In the PREMIER study, a behavioral intervention trial of 810 prehypertensive and hypertensive individuals, reduced sugar-sweetened beverages or sugar intake over 18 months was associated with reduced blood pressure [83].

Metabolic Syndrome / Insulin Resistance / Diabetes

Different definitions have been proposed for metabolic syndrome in the last few decades [84,85]. Metabolic syndrome is a combination of clinical and laboratory findings which include central adiposity, hypertension, dyslipidemia, inflammation, and impaired glucose tolerance that predispose affected individuals to atherosclerotic cardiovascular disease and Type 2 diabetes [84,86,87]. Insulin resistance is the key metabolic feature of metabolic syndrome [88].

Currently, epidemiological studies report an alarming worldwide increase in cardiovascular disease and metabolic syndrome [84]. Excessive fructose consumption in diet has been epidemiologically linked to the development of metabolic syndrome [89]. More recent findings suggest that high fructose intake induces a series of metabolic and cardiovascular alterations in both animal and human models [90]. However, there is a metabolic difference between rodents and primates, mainly in the lipoprotein metabolism, the main site for lipogenesis and the physiology of thermogenesis [88]. Increased dietary fructose intake in rats and dogs for several weeks has also shown many parameters of metabolic syndrome, including hypertension, insulin resistance, and hyperlipidemia [90]. The mechanism responsible for the adverse effects of fructose diet is not quite clear, but there is evidence that such a diet promotes gluco-oxidative stress.

Studies in rhesus monkeys have shown that fructose-sweetened drinks are well tolerated, and that within 6 to 12 months of consumption, a high-fructose diet produces many of the characteristics of metabolic syndrome in humans, including central obesity, insulin resistance, inflammation, and dyslipidemia [88]. High fructose consumption in humans increases ectopic fat deposition in the liver and skeletal muscle in young healthy individuals without a family history of diabetes [37] and increased hepatic inflammation and fibrosis [91]. Inflammation is a corollary of obesity, which is marked by a broad inflammatory response. Inflammation cytokine TNF-α is constitutively expressed in adipose tissue and over-expressed in rodent models of obesity [92]. Experimental studies have shown that fructose increases production of tumor necrosis factor (TNF-α), a pro-inflammatory cytokine which can induce peripheral resistance to insulin and production of lipoproteins [93].

Some studies have suggested a strong association between insulin resistance and endothelial dysfunction. Endothelial dysfunction induces vascular relaxation, with a reduction in the bioavailability of nitric oxide (NO) and an increase in oxidative stress and O_2^- superproduction levels, a key event for the development of cardiovascular complications associated to insulin resistance in experimental fructose-fed rat models [90].

Elderly, overweight, and obese patients were evaluated for fructose consumption and adverse effects. When fructose consumption corresponded to more than 25% of their energy needs, individuals presented increased visceral fat deposition and de novo lipogenesis, leading to dyslipidemia and reduced glucose tolerance [94]. Recent studies have reported that increased lipids is associated with increased diacylglycerol, which activates novel protein kinase C. Novel-PKC decreases tyrosine phosphorylation of the insulin receptor and/or insulin receptor substrate 1, resulting in increased hepatic glucose production, impaired glucose tolerance, and increased fasting glucose and insulin concentrations [84].

Fructose is also known to induce oxidative stress and mitochondrial dysfunction, resulting in the stimulation of peroxisome proliferator-activated receptor gamma coactivator 1-α and β (PGC1-α and PGC-1β) that drive both insulin resistance and lipogenesis [95,96]. The effect of fructose in lipogenesis has been reported as having the ability to alter the activity of key lipogenesis enzymes and transcription factors in the liver, such as pyruvate dehydrogenase kinase and sterol regulatory element-binding protein-1c (SREBP-1c), the main inducer of hepatic lipogenesis.

Conclusion

This chapter deals with the clinical and pathological aspects linked to high dietary fructose intake. The increase is specifically due to the introduction of HFCS as a sweetener in the United States, but less so in other parts of the world.

The adverse effects have been thoroughly demonstrated in experimental models, confirming the lipogenic effect of excessive fructose ingestion, with increased blood triglycerides, visceral lipids, insulin resistance, vascular dysfunction, and hypertension. However clinical studies, especially the epidemiological ones, associating the worldwide obesity epidemic [97], hypertension, and Type 2 diabetes to fructose, show several confounding factors and require better investigation.

Questions are raised in evaluating the studies; these include the amount of fructose ingested, diet duration, the previous presence of diabetes, and type of sweetener, remembering that HFCS and sucrose are similar in composition [98], Although free fructose is not in daily use, comparison between the effects of fructose and glucose have shown that the adverse effects are due to fructose [2]. Authors reported that the world obesity epidemic increases in the same proportion of sugar and sweeteners consumption. In addition, other authors have considered that fat consumption was reduced while obesity and fructose consumption increased in an epidemic manner [99]. Future studies can better elucidate the role of fructose in the pathophysiology of insulin resistance, metabolic syndrome, hypertension, and cardiac diseases.

References

[1] Henry, RR; Crapo, P; Thornburn, AN. Current issues in fructose metabolism. *Annu Rev Nutr,* 1991;11:21-39.

[2] Tappy, L; Lê, K-A. Metabolic effects of fructose and the worldwide increase in obesity. *Physiol Rev,* 2010;90:23-46.

[3] Mathews, RH; Pehrsson, PR; Farhat-Sabet, M (1987). Sugar content of selected foods: individual and total sugars. *Home Economics Research Report no 48,* Human Nutrition Information Service USDA. pp. 3-14. Government Printing Office, Washington, D.C.
[4] Marshall, RO; Koo, ER. Enzymatic conversion of D-glucose to D-fructose. *Science,* 1957;125:648-649.
[5] Bray, A; Nielsen, J; Popkin, BM. Consumption of high-fructose corn syrup in beverages may play a role in the epidemic of obesity. *Am J Clin Nutr Nutr,* 2004;79:537-43.
[6] Wang, YM; Van Eys, J. Nutritional significance of fructose and sugar alcohols. *Ann Rev Nutr,* 1981;1:437-75.
[7] Rumessen, JJ. Fructose and related food carbohydrates. *Scand J Gastroenterol,* 1992;27:819-828.
[8] Park, YK; Yetley, EA. Intakes and food sources of fructose in the United States. *Am J Clin Nutr,* 1993;58(Suppl):737S-747S.
[9] Brazilian Institute of Geography and Statistics. *Familiar Budget Survey,* 1996. URL: http://www.ibge.gov.br/ (portuguese).
[10] Perman, JA. Digestion and absorption of fruit juice carbohydrates. *J Am Coll Nutr,* 1996;15(5Suppl):S12-S17.
[11] Kneepkens, CMF; Vonk, RJ; Fernandes, J. Incomplete intestinal absorption of fructose. *Arch Dis Child,* 1984;59:735-738.
[12] Shi, X; Schedl, HP; Summers, RM; Lambert, GP; Chang, RT; Xia, T; Gisolfi, CV. Fructose transport mechanism in humans. *Gastroenterology,* 1997;113:1171-1179.
[13] Born, P.The clinical impact of carbohydrate malabsorption. *Arab J Gastroenterol,* 2011;12:1-4.
[14] Hallffrisch, J. Metabolic effects of dietary fructose. *FASEB J,* 1990;4:332-339.
[15] Koo, HY; Wallig, MA; Chung, BH; Nara, TY; Cho, BH; Nakamura, MT. Dietary fructose induces a wide range of genes with distinct shift in carbohydrates and lipid metabolism in fed and fasted rat liver. *Biochim Biophys Acta,* 2008;1782:341-348.
[16] Chong, MF-F; Fielding, BA; Frayn, KN. Mechanisms for acute effect of fructose on postprandial lipemia. *Am J Clin Nutr,* 2007;85:1511-1520.
[17] McGilvery, RW. Fructose Metabolism. In: *Biochemistry. A functional approach.* Philadelphia. London. Toronto; W.B. Saunders Company; 1970, Pg 631-634.
[18] Parks, JE; Hellerstein, MK. Carbohydrate-induced hypertriacyl-glycerolemia: historical perspective and review of biological mechanisms. *Am J Clin Nutr,* 2000;71:412-433.
[19] Tran, LT; Yuen, VG; McNeil, JH. The fructose-fed rat: a review on the mechanisms of fructose-induced insulin resistance and hypertension. *Mol Cell Biochem,* 2009;330:219-228.
[20] Schaefer, EJ; Gleason, JA; Dansinger, ML. Dietary fructose and glucose differentially affect lipid and glucose homeostasis. *J Nutr,* 2009;139:1257S-1262S.
[21] Topping, DL; Mayes, PA. The immediate effects of insulin and fructose on the metabolism of the perfused liver. Changes in lipoprotein secretion, fatty acid oxidation and esterification, and lipogenesis, and carbohydrate metabolism. *Biochem J,* 1972;126:295-311.
[22] Kasumi, T; Vranic, M; Steiner, G. Triglyceride kinetics: effects of dietary glucose, sucrose, or fructose alone or with hyperinsulinemia. *Am J Physiol Endocrinol Metab,* 1986;250:E325-E330.

[23] Froesch, ER. Disorders of fructose metabolism. *Clin Endocrinol Metab,* 1976;5:599-611.

[24] Clements, RS; Morrison, AD; Winegrad, AI. Polyol pathway in aorta. Regulation by hormones. *Science,* 1969;166:1007-1008.

[25] Setchell, BP; Bassett, JM; Hinks, NT; Graham, NMcC. The importance of glucose in the oxidative metabolism of the pregnant uterus and its contents in conscious sheep with some preliminary observations on the oxidation of fructose and glucose by fetal sheep. *Q J Exp Physiol,* 1972;57:257-266.

[26] Teng, CC; Tjoa, S; Fennessey, PV; Wilkening, RB; Battaglia, FC. Transplacental carbohydrate and sugar alcohol concentrations and their uptakes in ovine pregnancy. *Exp Biol Med,* 2002;227:189-195.

[27] Bossolan, G; Trindade, CEP; Barreiros, RC. Blood galactose and glucose levels in mothers, cord blood, and 48-hour-old breast-fed full-term infants. *Neonatology,* 2007;91:121-126.

[28] Jauniaux, E; Hempstock, J; Teng, C; Battaglia, FC; Burton, G. Polyol concentrations in fluid compartments of the human conceptus during the first trimester of pregnancy: maintenance of redox potential in a low oxygen environment. *J Clin Endocrinol Metab,* 2005;90:1171-1175.

[29] Brusati, V; Józwik, M; Teng, C; Paolini, C; Marconi, AM; Battaglia, FC. Fetal and maternal non-glucose carbohydrates and polyols concentrations in normal human pregnancies at term. *Pediatr Res,* 2006;58:700-704.

[30] Brachet, EA. Presence of the complete sorbitol pathway in the human normal umbilical cord tissue. *Biol Neonate*, 1973;23:314-323.

[31] Meznarich, HK; Hay Jr, W; Sparks, JW; Meschia, G; Battaglia. FC. Fructose disposal and oxidation rates in the ovine fetus. *Q J Exp Physiol,* 1987;72:617-625.

[32] Aeberli, I; Zimermann, MB; Molinari, L; Lehmann, R; L'Allemand, D; Spinas, GA; Berneis, K. Fructose intake is a predictor of LDL particle size in overweight schoolchildren. *Am J Clin Nutr,* 2007;86:1174-1178.

[33] Trindade, CEP; Barreiros, RC; Kurokawa, C; Bossolan, G. Fructose in fetal cord blood and its relationship with maternal and 48-hour-newborn blood concentrations. *Early Hum Dev,* 2011;87:193-197.

[34] Scott, TW; Setchell, B; Bassett, JM. Characterization and metabolism of ovine fetal lipids. *Biochem J,* 1967;104:1040-1047.

[35] Carmona, A; Freedland, RA. Comparison among the lipogenic potential of various substrates in rat hepatocytes: the differencial effects of fructose-containing diets on hepatic lipogenesis. *J Nutr,* 1989;119:1304-1310.

[36] Chico, A; D'Alessandro, ME; Karabatas, L; Pastorale, C; Basabe, JC; Lombardo, YB. Muscle lipid metabolism and insulin secretion are altered in insulin-resistant rats fed a high sucrose diet. *J Nutr,* 2003;133:127-133.

[37] Lê, K-A; Ith, M; Kreis, R; Faeh, D; Bortolotti, M; Tran, C; Boesch, C; Tappy, L. Fructose overconsumption causes dyslipidemia and ectopic lipid deposition in healthy subjects with and without a family history of type 2 diabetes. *Am J Clin Nutr,* 2009;89:1760-1765.

[38] Tappy, L; Lê, KA; Tran, C; Paquot N. Fructose and metabolic diseases: New findings, new questions. *Nutrition,* 2010;26:1044-1049.

[39] Jeukendrup, AE. Carbohydrate intake during exercise and performance. *Nutrition,* 2004;20:669-677.

[40] Adopo, E; Peronnet, F; Massicotte, D; Brisson, GR; Hillaire, C. Respective oxidation of exogenous glucose and fructose given in the same drink during exercise. *J Appl Physiol,* 1994;76:1014-1019.

[41] Jeukendrup, AE; Moseley, L; Mainwaring, GI; Samuels, S; Perry, S; Mann, CH. Exogenous carbohydrate oxidation during ultraendurance exercise. *J Appl Physiol,* 2006;100:1134-1141.

[42] Currell, K; Jeukendrup, AE. Superior endurance performance with ingestion of multiple transportable carbohydrates. *Med Sci Sports Exerc,* 2008;40:275-281.

[43] Bergman, BC; Wolfel, EE; Butterfield, GE; Lopaschuk, GD; Casazza, GA; Horning, MA; Brooks, GA. Active muscle and whole body lactate kinetics after endurance training in men. *J Appl Physiol*, 1999;87:1684-1696.

[44] Van Hall, G; Jensen-Urstad, M; Rosdahl, H; Holmberg, HC; Saltin, B; Calbet, JA. Leg and arm lactate and substrate kinetics during exercise. *Am J Physiol Endocrinol Metab,* 2003;284:E193-E205.

[45] LeCoutre, V; Benoit, R; Carrel, G; Schutz, Y; Millet, GP; Tappy, L; Schneiter, P. Fructose and glucose co-ingestion during prolonged exercise increases lactate and glucose fluxes and oxidation compared with an equimolar intake of glucose. *Am J Clin Nutr,* 2010;92:1071-1079.

[46] Stanhope, KL; Griffen, SC; Bair, BR; Swarbrick, MM; Keim, NL; Havel, PJ. Twenty-four-hour endocrine and metabolic profiles following consumption of high-fructose corn syrup-, sucrose-, fructose-, and glucose-sweetened beverages with meals. *Am J Clin Nutr,* 2008;87:1194-1203.

[47] Herman, RH; Zakim, D; Stifel FB. Effect of diet on lipid metabolism in experimental animals and man. *Fed Proc,* 1970;29:1302-1307.

[48] Havel, PJ. Dietary Fructose: Implications for dysregulation of energy homeostasis and lipid/carbohydrate metabolism. *Nutr Rev,* 2005;63:133-157.

[49] Bantle, JP; Raatz, SK; Thomas, W; Georgepoulos, A. Effects of dietary fructose on plasma lipids in healthy subjects. *Am J Clin Nutr,* 2000;72:1128-1134.

[50] Sievenpiper, JL; Carleton, AJ; Chatha S; Jiang, HY; De Souza, RJ; Beyene, J; Kendall, CWC; Jenkins, DJA. Heterogeneous effects of fructose on blood lipids in individuals with type 2 diabetes. *Diabetes Care*, 2009;32:1930-1937.

[51] Stanhope, KL; Bremer, AA; Medici, V; Nakajima, K; Ito, Y; Nakano, T; Chen, G; Fong, TH; Lee, V; Menorca, RI; Keim, NL; Havel, P. Consumption of fructose and high fructose corn syrup increase postprandial triglycerides, LDL-cholesterol, and apolipoprotein-B in young men and women. *J Clin Endocrinol Metab,* 2011;96:E1596-1605.

[52] Livesey, G; Taylor, R. Fructose consumption and consequences for glycation, plasma triacylglycerol, and body weight: meta-analyses and meta-regression models of intervention studies. *Am J Clin Nutr, 2008;88:1419-1437.*

[53] Marriott, BP; Cole, N; Lee, E. National estimates of dietary fructose intake increased from 1977 to 2004 in the United States. *J Nutr,* 2009;139:1228-1235.

[54] Elliott, SS; Keim, NL; Stern, JS; Teff, K; Havel, PJ. Fructose, weight gain, and the insulin resistance syndrome. *Am J Clin Nutr,* 2002;76:911-922.

[55] Swarbrick, MM; Stanhope, KL; Elliott, SS; Graham, JL; Krauss, RM; Christiansen, MP; Griffen, SC; Keim, NL; Havel P. Consumption of fructose-sweetened beverages for 10 weeks increases postprandial triacylglycerol and apolipoprotein-B concentrations in overweight and obese women. *Br J Nutr,* 2008;100:947-952.

[56] Aeberli, I; Zimmermann, MB; Molinari, L; Lehman, R; L'Allemand, D; Spinas, GA; Berneis, K. *Am J Nutr,* 2007;86:1174-1178.

[57] L'Allemand-Jander, D. Clinical diagnosis of metabolic and cardiovascular risks in overweight children; early development of chronic diseases in the obese child. *Int J Obes* (Lond), 2010;34(Suppl):S32-S36.

[58] Jürgens, H; Haass, W; Castañeda, TR; Schürmann, A; Koebnick, C; Dombrowski, F; Otto, B; Nawrocki, AR; Scherer, PE; Spranger, J; Ristow, M; Joost, H-G; Havel, PJ; Tschöp, H. Consuming fructose-sweetened beverages increases body adiposity in mice. *Obes Res,* 2005;13:1146-1156.

[59] Teff, KL; Elliott, SS; Tschop, M; Kieffer, TJ; Rader, D; Heiman, M; Townsend, RR; Keim, NL; D´Alessio, D; Havel, PJ. Dietary fructose reduces circulating insulin and leptin, attenuates postprandial suppression of ghrelin, and increases triglycerides in women. *J Clin Endocrinol Metab,* 2004;89:2963-2972.

[60] Stanhope, KL; Schwarz, JM; Keim, Nl; Griffen, SC; Bremer, AA; Graham, JL; Hatcher, B; Cox, CL; Dyachenko, A; Zhang, W; Mc Graham, JL; Seibert, A; Kraus, RM; Chiu, S; Schaefer, EJ; Ai, M; Otokozawa, S; Nakajima, K; Nakano, T; Beysen, C; Hellerstein, MK; Berglund, L; Havel, PJ. Consuming fructose-sweetened, not glucose-sweetened beverages increases visceral adiposity and lipids and decreases insulin sensitivity in overweight/obese humans. *J Clin Invest,* 2009;119:1322-1334.

[61] Bantle, JP; Laine, DC; Castle, GW; Thomas, JW; Hoogvert, BJ; Goetz, FC. Postprandial glucose and insulin responses to meals containing different carbohydrates in normal and diabetic subjects. *N Engl J Med,* 1983;309:7-12

[62] Havel, PJ. Control of energy homeostasis and insulin action by adipocyte hormones: leptin, acylation stimulating protein, and adiponectin. *Curr Opin Lipidol,* 2002;13:51-59.

[63] .Teff, KL; Grudziak, J; Townsend, RB; Dunn, TN; Grant, RW; Adams, SH; Keim, NL; Cummings, BP; Stanhope, KL; Havel, PJ. Endocrine and metabolic effects of consuming fructose- and glucose-sweetened beverages with meals in obese men and women: influence of insulin resistance on plasma triglyceride responses. *J Clin Endocrinol Metab,* 2009;94:1562-1569.

[64] Cirillo, P; Sato, W; Reungjui, S; Heinig, M; Gersch, M; Sautin, Y; Nakagawa, T; Johnson, RJ. Uric acid, the metabolic syndrome, and renal disease. *J Am Soc Nephrol,* 2006;17(12 Suppl 3):S165-S168.

[65] Johnson, RJ; Perez-Pozo, SE; Sautin, YY; Manitius, J; Sanchez-Lozada, LG; Feig, DI; Shafiu, M; Segal, M; Glassock, RJ; Shimada, M; Roncal, C; Nakagawa, T. Hypothesis: could excessive fructose intake and uric acid cause type 2 diabetes? *Endocr Rev,* 2009;30:96-116.

[66] Johnson, RJ; Sanchez-Lozada, LG; Nakagawa, T. The effect of fructose on renal biology and disease. *J Am Soc Nephrol,* 2010;21:2036-2039.

[67] Nakagawa, T; Hu, H; Zharikov, S; Tuttle, KR; Short, RA; Glushakova, O; Ouyang, X; Feig, DI; Block, ER; Herrera-Acosta, J; Patel, JM; Johnson, RJ. A causal role for uric acid in fructose-induced metabolic syndrome. *Am J Physiol Renal Physiol,* 2006;290:F625-F631.

[68] Graessler, J; Graessler, A; Unger, S; Kopprasch, S; Tausche, AK; Kuhlisch, E; Schroeder, HE; Feig, DI; Johnson, RJ. The role of uric acid in pediatric hypertension. *J Ren Nut,* 2007;17:79-83.

[69] Feig, DD; Johnson RJ. The role of uric acid in pediatric hypertension. *J Ren Nutr,* 2007;17:79-83.

[70] Khosla, UM; Zharikov, S; Finch, JL; Nakagawa, T; Roncal, C; Mu, W; Krotova, K; Block, ER; Prabhakar, S; Johnson, RJ. Hyperuricemia induces endothelial dysfunction. *Kidney Int,* 2005;67:1739-1742.

[71] Bunag, RD; Tomita, T; Sasaki, S. Chronic sucrose ingestion induces mild hypertension and tachycardia in rats. *Hypertension,* 1983;5:218-225.

[72] Martinez, FJ; Rizza, RA; Romero, JC. High-fructose feeding elicits insulin resistance, hyperinsulinism, and hypertension in normal mongrel dogs. *Hypertension,* 1994;23: 456-463.

[73] Kamide, K; Rakugi, H; Higaki, J; Okamura, A; Nagai, M; Moriguchi, K; Ohishi, M; Satoh, N; Tuck, ML; Ogihara, T. The rennin-angiotensin and adrenergic nervous system in cardiac hypertrophy in fructose-fed rats. *Am J Hypertens,* 2002;15:66-71.

[74] Miller, AW; Sims, JJ; Canavan, A; Hsu, T; Ujhelyi, MR. Impaired vagal reflex activity in insulin-resistance rats. *J Cardiovasc Pharmacol,* 1999;33:698-702.

[75] Sanchez-Lozada, LG; Tapia, E; Jimenez, A; Bautista, P; Cristobal, M; Nepomuceno, T; Soto, V; Avila-Casado, C; Nakagawa, T; Johnson, RJ; Herrero-Acosta, J; Franco, M. Fructose-induced metabolic syndrome is associated with glomerular hypertension and renal microvascular damage in rats. *Am J Physiol Renal Physiol,* 2007;292:F423-F429.

[76] Brown, CM; Dulloo, AG; Yepuri, G; Montani, JP. Fructose ingestion acutely elevates blood pressure in healthy young humans. *Am J Physiol Regul Integr Comp Physiol,* 2008;294:R730-R737.

[77] Brown, IJ; Stamler, J; Van Horn, L; Robertson, CE; Chan, Q; Dyer, AR; Huang, C-C; Rodriguez, BL; Zhao, L; Daviglus, ML; Ueshima, H; Elliott, P. International Study of Macro/Micronutrients and Blood Pressure Research Group. Sugar-Sweetened Beverage, Sugar Intake of Individuals, and their Blood Pressure International Study of Macro/Micronutrients and Blood Pressure. *Hypertension,* 2011;57:695-701.

[78] Johnson, RJ; Segal, MS; Sautin, Y; Takahiko, N; Feig, DI; Kang, DH; Gersch, MS; Benner, S; Sánchez-Lozada, L. Potential role of sugar (fructose) in the epidemic of hypertension, obesity and the metabolic syndrome, diabetes, kidney disease, and cardiovascular disease. *Am J Clin Nutr,* 2007;86:899-906.

[79] Mazzali, M; Kanellis, J; Han, L; Feng, L; Xia, YY; Chen, Q; Kang, DH; Gordon, KL; Watanabe, S; Nakagawa, T; Lan, HY; Johnson RJ. Hyperuricemia induces a primary renal arteriolopathy in rats by a blood pressure-independent mechanism. *Am J Physiol Renal Physiol,* 2002;282:F991-F997.

[80] Watanabe, S; Kang, DH; Feng, L; Nakagawa, T; Kanellis, J; Lan, H; Mazzali, M; Johnson, RJ. Uric acid, hominoid evolution and the pathogenesis of salt-sensivity. *Hypertension,* 2002:40:355-60.

[81] Quiroz, Y; Pons, H; Gordon, KL; Rincón, J; Chávez, M; Parra, G; Herrera-Acosta, J. Mycophenolate mofetil prevents salt-sensitivite hypertension resulting from nitric synthesis inhibition. *Am J Physiol Renal Physiol,* 2001;281:F38-F47.
[82] Soleimani, M. Dietary fructose, salt absorption and hypertension in metabolic syndrome: towards a new paradigm. *Acta Physiol,* 2011;201:55-62.
[83] Chen, L; Caballero, B; Mitchell, DC; Loria, C; Lin, P-H; Champagne, CM; Elmer, PJ; Ard, JD; Batch, BC; Anderson, CAM; Appel, LJ. Reducing consumption of sugar-sweetened beverages is associated with reduced blood pressure: a prospective study among United States adults. *Circulation,* 2010;121:2398-2406.
[84] Meigs, JB. Epidemiology of type 2 diabetes and cardiovascular disease: translation from population to prevention: The Kelly West award lecture, 2009. *Diabetes Care,* 2010;33:1865-1871.
[85] Alberti, KG; Zimmet, P; Shaw, J. The metabolic syndrome: a new worldwide definition. IDF Epidemiology Task Force Consensus Group. *Lancet,* 2005; **366:**1059-1062.
[86] Antonoupolos, S. National Cholesterol Education Program (NCEP) Expert Panel on Detection, Evaluation, and treatment of High Blood Cholesterol in Adults (Adult Treatment Panel III). Third Report of the National Cholesterol Education (NCEP) Expert Panel on Detection, Evaluation, and treatment of High Blood Cholesterol in Adults (Adult Treatment Panel III) final report. *Circulation,* 2002;106:3143-3421.
[87] Grundy, SM; Cleeman, JI; Daniels, SR; Donato, KA; Eckel, RH; Franklin, BA; Gordon, DJ; Krauss, RM; Savage, PJ; Smith Jr, SC; Spectus, JA; Costa, F. Diagnosis and management of the metabolic syndrome: an American Heart Association/National Heart, Lung, and Blood Institute Scientific Statement. *Circulation,* 2005;**112:**2735-2752 [published corrections appear in Circulation 2005;112:e297 and Circulation 2005;112:e298].
[88] Bremer, AA; Stanhope, KL; Graham, BS; Cummings, BP; Wang, W; Saville, BR; Havel, PJ. Fructose-Fed Rhesus Monkeys: A Nonhuman Primate Model of Insulin Resistance, Metabolic Syndrome, and Type 2 Diabetes. *Clin Trans Sci,* 2011; 4:243-252.
[89] Collino, M. High dietary fructose intake: sweet or bitter life? *World J Diabetes,* 2011;15:77-81.
[90] Korandji, C; Zeller, M; Guilland, JC; Collin, B; Lauzier, B; Sicard, P; Duvillard, L; Goirand, F; Moreau, D; Cottin, Y; Rochette, L; Vergel, YC. Time course of asymmetric dimethylarginine (ADMA) and oxidative stress in fructose-hypertensive rats: A model related to metabolic syndrome. *Atherosclerosis,* 2011;214:310-315.
[91] Abdelmalek, MF; Suzuki, A; Guy, C; Unalp-Arida; A; Colvin, R; Johnson, RJ; Diehl, AM. Increased fructose consumption is associated with fibrosis severity in patients with nonalcoholic fatty liver disease. *Hepatology* 2010; 51:1961-1971.
[92] Pradhan, A. Obesity, Metabolic Syndrome, and Type 2 Diabetes: Inflammatory Basis of Glucose Metabolic Disorders. *Nutr Rev,* 2007;65: S152-156.
[93] Kanuri, G; Spruss, A; Wagnerberger, S; Bischoff, SC; Bergheim, I. Role of tumor necrosis factor α (TNFα) in the onset of fructose-induced nonalcoholic fatty liver disease in mice. *J Nutr Biochem,* 2011; 22: 527-534.
[94] Stanhope, KL. Role of Fructose-Containing Sugars in the Epidemics of Obesity and Metabolic Syndrome. *Annu Rev Med,* 2011; Jan 26. [Epub ahead of print].

[95] Nagai, Y; Yonemitsu, S; Erion, DM; Iwasaki, T; Stark, R; Weismann, D; Dong, J; Zhang, D; Jurczak, MJ; Löffler, MG; Cresswell, J; Yu, XX; Murray, SF; Bhanot, S; Monia, BP; Bogan, JS; Samuel, V; Shulman, GI. The role of peroxisome proliferator-activated receptor gamma coactivator-1 beta in the pathogenesis of fructose-induced insulin resistance. *Cell Metab,* 2009;9: 252-264.

[96] Lin, J; Handschin, C; Spiegelman, BM. Metabolicc control through the PGC-1 family of transcription coativators. *Cell Metab,* 1: 361-370, 2005.

[97] White, S. Straight talk about high-fructose corn syrup: what it is and what it ain't. *Am J Clin Nutr*, 2008;88(Suppl):1716S-1721S.

[98] Wiernsperger, N; Geloen, A; Rapin, J-R. Fructose and cardiometabolic disorders: The controversy will, and must, continue. *Clinics*, 2010;65:729-738.

[99] Johnson, RJ; Segal, S M; Sautin, Y; Nakagawa, T; Feig, DI; Kang, D-H; Gersch, MS; Benner, S; Sánchez-Lozada, LG. Potential role of sugar (fructose) in the epidemic of hypertension, obesity and the metabolic syndrome, diabetes, kidney disease, and cardiovascular disease. *Am J Clin Nutr,* 2007;86:899-906.

In: Fructose
Editors: Brandon M. Johnston and Aaron B. Collins ISBN: 978-1-62081-126-9

Chapter 3

FRUCTOSE AND NON-ALCOHOLIC FATTY LIVER DISEASE

Ting Zhang[1], Shen Qu[2], Steven Ringquist[1], and H. Henry Dong[1*]

[1] Rangos Research Center, Division of immunogenetics,
Department of Pediatrics, Children's Hospital of Pittsburgh,
University of Pittsburgh School of Medicine, Pittsburgh, Pennsylvania, US
[2] Shanghai Tenth People's Hospital ,
Tongji University School of Medicine, Shanghai, PR, China

ABSTRACT

Fructose is referred to as fruit sugar that is highly enriched in corn syrup. High fructose corn syrup is increasingly used as a sweetener in processed foods, baked goods, and carbonated soft drinks. High consumption of fructose is alleged as a causative factor for non-alcoholic fatty liver disease, a pathological condition that is characterized by excessive fat accumulation in the liver of individuals who drink little or no alcohol. It is puzzling as to how chronic consumption of refined fructose in carbonated beverages is associated with adverse effects, whereas daily intake of fructose-containing fruits and honey is considered beneficial for health. In this chapter, we will review the molecular mechanism by which fructose is metabolized in the body and provide unbiased view of whether fructose consumption is a risk factor for nonalcoholic fatty liver disease.

Keywords: Fructose, Non-Alcoholic Fatty Liver Disease, Metabolic Syndrome, Insulin Resistance, Hypertriglyceridemia, Type 2 Diabetes.

---

[*] Correspondence should be addressed to: Dr. Dong Rangos Research Center, Children's Hospital of Pittsburgh, 530 45th Street, Rm 6124, Pittsburgh, PA 15201, Tel: +1 (412) 692-6324, Fax: +1 (412) 692-5809, Email: dongh @pitt.edu

INTRODUCTION

Beginning in the 1970s, there has been a dramatic increase in obesity. Today, approximately 68% of adults in the U.S. are overweight, 33.8% of these individuals are obese with nearly 5.7% of American adults severely obese [1]. An increasingly growing concern is the prevalence of childhood obesity. Over the same time period, the prevalence of childhood obesity has more than doubled for preschool children aged 2-5 years (5.0% to 10.4%), aged 6-11 (6.5% to 19.6%) and tripled among adolescents aged 12-19 years (5.0 to 18.1%). About nine million children are considered obese having BMI values at or above the 95 percentile of age and gender matched cohorts. Obesity is a predisposing factor for metabolic syndrome that is characterized by abnormal glucose and lipid metabolism. Obesity greatly compromises the quality of life, accompanied by decreased self-esteem and increased depression. When left unabated, obesity consequently leads to fatty liver disease, sleep apnea, hypertension, insulin resistance and diabetes. Morbid obesity has become the second leading cause of preventable death in the U.S. Apart from genetic predisposition and sedentary life style, factors that contribute to the obesity epidemic remain elusive.

Based on epidemiologic studies of obesity in relation to increased per capital consumption of high fructose corn syrup (HFCS) from beverages, excessive dietary intake of fructose is alleged as a confounding factor for the increased prevalence of overweight and morbid obesity [2]. There is evidence that frequent consumption of sugar-sweetened soft drinks is a potential contributing factor for childhood obesity [3-6]. Fructose, which occurs naturally in honey and sweet fruits, is produced in crystalline and syrup forms for commercial use. The most commonly used corn syrup contains about 55% free fructose (HFCS-55, used commonly in beverages) or 42% free fructose (HFCS-42, used commonly in processed food or baked goods), and its use as a sweetener in processed foods and soft drinks has greatly increased by 20-30% over the past 20 years, a rate of increase in par with the incidence of obesity that has risen dramatically over the same period of time [2, 7-9]. Such a seemingly linear correlation between increased consumption of fructose and bourgeoning prevalence of obesity is both disturbing and puzzling. While daily intake of fructose-containing fruits and honey is considered beneficial for health, chronic consumption of refined fructose in carbonated beverages is associated with adverse effects. This begets the question: why is fructose, as opposed to other sugars, particularly deleterious to metabolism? In this article, we review the distinct mechanism by which fructose is metabolized in the body and provide insightful discussion on how excessive fructose consumption perturbs normal glucose and lipid metabolism. While the global effect of excessive fructose intake on health in animal models and humans has been reviewed elsewhere [9-12], we focus our review on the liver to address the fundamental question of how sustained fructose consumption contributes to the development of insulin resistance and non-alcoholic fatty liver disease (NAFLD).

FRUCTOSE CATABOLISM IN THE LIVER

There is emerging evidence that increased fructose consumption is a causative factor for non-alcoholic fatty liver disease, a pathological condition that is characterized by increased fat deposition in the liver of individuals who drink little or no alcohol (less than 10 grams of alcohol per day for women and less than 20 grams per pay for men, or the equivalent of less than 1 and 2 standard drinks per day for women and men, respectively). This effect is exacerbated by prevailing health conditions such as obesity and type 2 diabetes. To comprehend the underlying mechanism, we need to understand the metabolic pathway in which fructose is catablized in the body. Fructose breakdown takes place mainly in the liver in a metabolic pathway that is different from glucose metabolism in three fundamental ways.

First, after its absorption in the gastrointestinal track, fructose present in the portal blood is rapidly extracted by the liver [13]. The liver is responsible for metabolic uptake of the bulk of absorbed fructose [9, 14-16]. Unlike glucose that enters the liver through glucose transporter 2 (Glut2) that is stimulated by insulin, fructose enters hepatocytes via glucose transporter 5 (Glut5) independently of insulin action [17]. Second, fructose, as opposed to glucose, does not directly stimulate pancreatic insulin release, due to the lack of Glut5 expression in pancreatic beta cells [17]. Postprandial insulin secretion is instrumental for modulating glucose metabolism in peripheral tissues and regulating energy balance via the central nervous system through both direct and indirect mechanisms to control food intake and body weight gain [18-21]. However, such an energy balancing mechanism does not respond to dietary fructose uptake, due to the inability of fructose to elicit insulin release. Third, glucose metabolism is negatively regulated by phosphofructokinase, a hepatic enzyme that regulates glycolysis in the liver. In contrast, fructose is metabolized into glycerol-3-phosphate and acetyl-CoA, bypassing this rate-limiting feedback control mechanism. As a result, increased fructose influx to the liver results in massive production of glycerol-3-phosphate and acetyl-CoA, two intermediate metabolites that are substrates for triglyceride synthesis, contributing to increased very low-density lipoprotein (VLDL)-triglyceride (TG) production in the liver [22, 23]. Prior to dissecting the molecular mechanism underlying fructose-induced fatty liver disease, we would like to review the evidence regarding the impact of fructose on body mass and hormonal responses to illustrate how excessive fructose consumption can favor energy storage and promote ectopic fat accumulation, a major risk factor for the development of insulin resistance and type 2 diabetes.

Fructose Consumption and Its Impact on Body Mass

A variety of studies have linked fructose overconsumption to increased body mass. For example, in a study of 548 schoolchildren followed over a time period of 2 academic years (Grades 6 and 7), the mean body mass index (BMI) increases by 0.18 kg/m^2 with each daily serving, and by 0.24 kg/m^2 with each additional serving of sugar sweetened drink [3]. Likewise, a study performed on a cohort of 103 adolescents (ages 13 to 18 years) indicated that reduction in the consumption of sugar-sweetened beverage also reduced BMI, especially among obese subjects [24]. These observations have been recapitulated in animal studies. In studies involving mice, feeding with fructose also increases body mass, with similar results reported for hamsters and dogs [22, 23, 25, 26]. Fructose intake as well as obesity has been linked with increased risk of type 2 diabetes [27, 28].

The National Health and Nutrition Examination Survey (NHANES) [29] has estimated that nearly 68% of adults in the U.S. are overweight (BMI > 25 kg/m^2) and 33.8% are classified as obese (BMI > 30 kg/m^2). Among children and adolescents, 16.9% are obese with the prevalence of obesity higher among non-Hispanic black males (19.8%) and Mexican-American males (26.8%) compared with non-Hispanic white adolescent males (16.7%). Similar trends were observed among adolescent females (non-Hispanic black, 29.2%; Mexican-American, 17.4%; and non-Hispanic white, 14.5%). Environmental factors appear to have a greater relative influence on rapid weight gain than are accounted for by known genetic variants [30-32]. Among the environmental factors impacting undue weight gain are overeating and physical inactivity. These behaviors may be of recent origin [33]. It is likely that during human history, the environment is typified by periods of frequent famine rather than the westernized lifestyle of food abundance and sedentary behavior. For example, studies of adolescents and young adults (ages 15 to 18) have indicated that this population consumes about 9.9% of caloric energy in the form of sugar from beverages [34].

EFFECT OF FRUCTOSE ON INSULIN SENSITIVITY:

Excessive fructose consumption contributes to insulin resistance, culminating in the development of hyperinsulinemia and glucose intolerance. This finding is persistently reproduced in animal models with high fructose feeding as well as in human subjects with overconsumption of fructose-sweetened beverages for a limited period of time. For example, Stanhope and colleagues determined the effect of glucose- versus fructose-sweetened beverages on weight gain and energy homeostasis in overweight and obese subjects [35]. They report that sustained consumption of fructose, but not glucose, containing beverages for 10 weeks results in significantly impaired glucose tolerance, elevated fasting blood glucose and plasma insulin levels. When compared to those consuming glucose-sweetened beverages, subjects consuming fructose-sweetened beverages also exhibit significantly increased visceral adiposity [35].

What is the underlying mechanism of fructose-induced insulin resistance? A simplest explanation is that insulin resistance is secondary to fructose-induced ectopic fat accumulation. In support of this notion, increased fat accumulation is detectable in the liver of animals with *ad libitum* drinking of fructose-containing water or fed a high fructose diet [35, 36]. It is generally conceived that hepatic fat infiltration is a predisposing factor for inducing insulin resistance [26, 37]. Nevertheless, it remains unclear whether hepatic fat accumulation precedes the development of insulin resistance.

To account for the mechanism of fructose-induced insulin resistance, Adeli and colleagues studied the effect of fructose feeding on the expression of protein-tyrosine phosphatase-1B (PTP1B), a negative regulator of insulin signaling [38]. They detect a significant induction of PTP1B protein mass and activity in the liver, correlating with the development of hepatic insulin resistance in hamsters after 4-week high fructose feeding [38]. This is reflected in the reduction of insulin-stimulated Akt-Ser473 and Akt-Thr308 phosphorylation in the liver of high fructose-fed hamsters [38]. Similar results of fructose-induced attenuation of Akt phosphorylation are produced in high fructose-fed rats [39]. Pharmacological inhibition of PTP1B activity improves lipid metabolism and prevents steatosis in fructose-fed rats [40].

In another study, Bezerra et al. [41] investigate the effect of fructose feeding on the early steps of insulin action in muscle and liver of rats. There are no differences in insulin receptor

(IR) and insulin receptor substrate 1 (IRS-1) protein levels in the liver and muscle of rats fed the control versus high fructose diets for 28 days. However, tyrosine-phosphorylation of IR and IRS-1 is significantly attenuated in both the liver and skeletal muscle in response to insulin stimulation in high fructose-fed rats [41], bolstering the idea that fructose feeding elicits insulin resistance.

To gain insight into the underlying mechanism of fructose-mediated hepatic insulin resistance, Wei and Pagliassotti demonstrate that intraportal fructose infusion, which raises portal vein fructose concentration to approximately 1 mM, results in a significant induction of hepatic JNK activity within 6 hours [42, 43]. This acute effect correlates with an impaired ability of insulin to stimulate IRS phosphorylation in fructose-treated livers. Furthermore, normalization of JNK activity in hepatocytes isolated from high fructose-fed rats improves insulin-stimulated tyrosine phosphorylation of IRS protein [42, 43]. Their studies unveil a mechanistic interplay between the activation of JNK stress pathway via Fructose-1-phosphatase activation of MKK7 (mitogen-activated protein kinase kinase 7) and subsequent stimulation of MAPK8 (mitogen-activated protein kinase 8) activity resulting in the onset of hepatic insulin resistance in fructose-fed rats [42, 44, 45].

Impact of Fructose on Leptin Signaling

Leptin is well-characterized adipose-derived hormone with central and peripheral effects on food intake and dietary substrate handling [46]. It regulates adiposity by decreasing food intake and increasing energy expenditure [47]. In humans, excessive obesity has been correlated with lack of leptin production [48] as well as loss of leptin-dependent cellular signaling [49]. In contrast, administration of exogenous leptin to a child with congenital leptin deficiency has been observed to decrease body mass [50]. Leptin treatment is seen to ameliorate metabolic abnormalities in patients with relative leptin deficiency due to lipoatrophy [51, 52].

Leptin secretion is linked to energy uptake though the interaction of insulin with glucose availability. In a recent study involving 17 obese individuals (BMI >30 kg/m^2), Teff et al. [53] compared the effect of glucose- versus fructose-sweetened beverage consumed with meals on leptin secretion. Fructose, as opposed to glucose, sweetened beverage is associated with relatively lower plasma leptin levels, accompanied by increased plasma triglyceride levels [35, 53]. Thus, similar to the inert effect of fructose on insulin release, fructose feeding does not stimulate leptin secretion [35, 53, 54].

Leptin is produced in adipose tissue and is subject to insulin regulation. In response to postprandial insulin secretion, leptin production is up-regulated through insulin-mediated alterations in glucose metabolism in adipose tissues [55, 56]. This effect acts in the central nervous system to suppress hunger and limit food intake [18, 19, 57]. However, such a feed-back control mechanism is impaired in response to fructose feeding, due to the inability of fructose to elicit insulin secretion. In fact, rats fed high fructose diets exhibited leptin resistance as indicated by loss of the anorectic effect of intraperitoneally administered leptin [58].

Fructose-induced leptin resistance has been linked with decreased phosphorylation of hypothalamic signal transducer and activator of transcription 3 (STAT3) [58] as well as hepatic STAT3 and suppressor of cytokine signaling-3 (SOC3), signal transducers that enhance fat mobilization and oxidation [59]. Moreover, the absence of fructose transporter GLUT5 in insulin-producing pancreatic beta cells is likely responsible for the lack of fructose-mediated insulin secretion [17].

When compared with glucose-containing drinks, consumption of fructose-sweetened beverages results in lower glucose, insulin, and leptin in circulation [60]. As a result, the combined effect of lower plasma insulin and leptin levels translates into a hunger signal to enhance food uptake, accompanied by fructose consumption. This is one of the reasons underlying the association between fructose overconsumption and increased incidence of obesity and subsequent diabetes [35, 53].

Impact of Fructose on Ghrelin Secretion

Ghrelin is regarded as a hunger hormone. Consistent with its role in regulating appetite, plasma ghrelin levels increase before meals and decrease after meals [61-64]. Ghrelin is produced mainly in the stomach [65, 66], and to a lesser extent in other organs such as the bowel [67], pituitary gland [68], kidney [69], placenta [70], and hypothalamus [65]. Ghrelin is also a secretagogue with a potent action to stimulate growth hormone release from anterior pituitary gland [71-76]. In rodents treated with ghrelin, excess food intake results in increased adiposity [62, 64, 77-81]. In humans, evidence for regulation of appetite by ghrelin has been provided by studies of a cohort of healthy volunteers, showing that three quarters of the participants exhibit hunger following administration of ghrelin [82]. This is confirmed by subsequent studies in which participants reported hunger in response to ghrelin exposure [83]. Ghrelin stimulation promotes food intake in human subjects [63] and animal models [84]. Studies in humans indicate that circulating ghrelin is positively correlated with obesity [61] and acute food intake [85].

Interestingly, there are increased ghrelin levels in serum after fructose feeding [86]. Although the underlying mechanism remains to be determined, the induction of ghrelin, resulting from fructose consumption, accounts in part for increased appetite and overeating. This effect also contributes to body weight gain [60].

Fructose Consumption and Hepatic Inflammation

There is evidence that increased fructose consumption is associated with hepatic inflammation. Increased plasma concentration of TNF-α has been observed in fructose-fed rodents [87, 88]. Furthermore, increased TNF-α mRNA levels are detectable in liver of fructose-fed mice [87, 89, 90]. Similarly, rats fed fructose-enriched diet also exhibit signify-cantly elevated levels of monocyte chemoattractant protein-1 (MCP-1) in liver [91]. In response to fructose feeding, the classical inflammatory NF-κB pathway is activated, which in turn contributes to hepatic inflammation [88, 92]. Hepatic inflammation exerts a direct impact on hepatic and intestinal secretion of lipoproteins. For example, *in vivo* TNF-α infusion for 4 h in hamsters significantly attenuates insulin-stimulated tyrosine phosphoryl-ation of insulin receptor (IR) and insulin receptor substrate-1 (IRS-1) and Akt, accompanied by excessive VLDL-TG production in liver [93]. Likewise, acute TNF-α infusion also decreases tyrosine phosphorylation of insulin receptor, IRS-1, and Akt in the intestine, leading to increased secretion of apoB48-containing chylomicrons [94]. To further illustrate the role of TNF-α in the pathogenesis of fructose-induced NAFLD, Kanuri and colleagues show that genetic depletion of the TNF-α receptor (TNFR1) protects against fructose-induced hepatic inflammation and steatosis in mice [95]. Together these data implicate hepatic inflammation as a significant risk factor for the development of insulin resistance and dyslipidemia in subjects with excessive fructose intake.

HIGH FRUCTOSE CONSUMPTION AND CARDIOVASCULAR DISEASE

Carbonated soft drinks supply roughly one-third of the world's daily sugar intake [96] and fructose is roughly one-half of the total sugar in soft drinks. In studies performed on dogs, fructose enriched diets have been linked with hypertension, elevated plasma triglycerides, insulin resistance, and hyperinsulemia [97]. The health effects associated with diets high in fructose have been reported by multiple clinical and preclinical studies. Overall, the available data support the hypothesis that excessive diet of fructose may contribute to increased blood pressure and related cardiovascular disease [57, 80, 98, 99]. Recent studies by Brown et al. [100] indicate that fructose ingestion acutely elevates blood pressure in humans. Their studies involve 15 healthy adults (aged 21-33 years), who consume 0.5 liters of fructose-sweetened drinks. When compared with ingestion of an equal volume of water, ingesting fructose drink significantly raises blood pressure, heart rate, and cardiac output for the ensuing 2 hours. Glucose ingestion also results in a significantly greater increase in cardiac output but without significant alterations in blood pressure. These data support the idea that fructose, rather than glucose, is the more damaging sugar component in terms of cardiovascular risk [101].

However, the molecular basis that links fructose feeding to cardiovascular risk is poorly understood and several studies have reported conflicting results correlating fructose feeding with hypertension [9]. It is likely multifactorial. Aside from fructose-elicited insulin resistance, fructose overconsumption results in the development of hypertriglyceridemia, a lipid disorder that is characterized by augmented production and/or retarded clearance of triglyceride-rich particles such as very low-density lipoproteins (VLDL) and chylomicrons [102-104]. This is consistently observed in human subjects with excessive fructose consumption for a limited period of time [35, 53, 60] and in animals fed a fructose-enriched diet [23, 26, 105-107]. Hypertriglyceridemia is an important component of metabolic syndrome and is a major risk factor for coronary artery disease.

To account for the underlying mechanisms, several independent studies show that fructose-fed hamsters exhibit markedly increased production of apolipoprotein B (ApoB) and microsomal triglyceride transfer protein (MTP, encoded by the MTTP gene) [26, 106, 108-111]. ApoB is the core component of VLDL and is responsible for VLDL assembly in the liver [112] and individuals heterozygous for premature truncation mutations in ApoB exhibit reduced levels of VLDL particles and nearly 3-fold increase in hepatic fat content [113]. MTP is regarded as a molecular chaperone that catalyzes the transfer of lipid to nascent apolipoprotein B (apoB), a rate-limiting step in hepatic VLDL production [114-116]. More recently, Qu et al. [23] demonstrate that high fructose feeding results in hepatic over-production of apolipoprotein C-III (apoC-III). ApoC-III functions as an inhibitor of lipoprotein lipase (LPL), a key enzyme in the hydrolysis of triglyceride in VLDL and chylomicrons [117, 118]. ApoC-III also inhibits hepatic lipase activity [119]. This effect, along with the induction of MTP and apoB production, results in impaired clearance of triglyceride-rich particles in plasma and augmented production of VLDL in the liver, contributing to the development of hypertriglyceridemia in high fructose-fed animals [25, 110, 120-122].

To delineate the mechanistic linkage between fructose overconsumption and the pathogenesis of hypertriglyceridemia, Qu et al. [23] studied the effect of fructose metabolism on FoxO1, a nuclear transcription factor that plays a key role in integrating insulin signaling to target gene expression in insulin sensitive tissues. FoxO1 comprises two structural domains, the amino forkhead domain that is necessary for DNA binding and the carboxyl *trans*-activation domain that is responsible for stimulating promoter activity [123]. Their studies show that FoxO1 targets both MTTP and ApoC-III genes for *trans*-activation [109, 120]. In response to high fructose feeding, FoxO1 activity is upregulated, which in turn promotes MTP and ApoC-III overproduction, contributing to increased secretion of VLDL from the liver and decreased clearance of triglyceride-rich particles in plasma. These data shed light on the etiology of hypertriglyceridemia in response to excessive fructose consumption, suggesting that FoxO1 dysregulation in the liver accounts in part for the development of hypertriglyceridemia [110]. FoxO1 may be a therapeutic target for improving triglyceride metabolism in obesity and type 2 diabetes.

In addition to its impact on triglyceride metabolism, fructose seems to exert an independent effect on cholesterol metabolism. Stanhope et al. [35] show that human subjects consuming fructose-sweetened beverages are associated with significantly higher plasma levels of small dense low-density lipoprotein (LDL), a proatherogenic profile that can predispose at-risk individuals to developing coronary artery disease over time. However, there is a lack of concrete evidence that high fructose consumption causes atherosclerosis. This is due in part to the fact that previous clinical trials involve a relatively short-term exposure (10 weeks) to fructose-enriched beverages and previous preclinical studies employ animal models that are genetically insusceptible to atherosclerosis. Thus, further investigation is warranted to determine whether prolonged overconsumption of fructose, as opposed to glucose, triggers the onset and promotes the progression of atherosclerosis in atherogenic animal models.

Association of Fructose Consumption with Non-Alcoholic Fatty Liver Disease

Nonalcoholic fatty liver disease (NAFLD) refers to a spectrum of liver disease that is characterized by excessive fat accumulation in hepatocytes. The term "nonalcoholic" is used because NAFLD occurs in individuals who do not usually consume a large amount of alcohol. NAFLD is the most common liver disease, affecting about 20% of the US population. However, larger estimates of hepatic steatosis have been reported in select regions of the country with, for example, Dallas County exhibiting an estimated 34% prevalence [1, 124]. When left unabated, NAFLD consequently advances to nonalcoholic steatohepatitis (NASH) and cirrhosis. To date, the underlying cause and mechanism of NAFLD still remains obscure.

It is noteworthy that excessive fructose consumption results in NAFLD. Such a metabolic mishap is consistently observed in a variety of animal models fed a fructose-enriched diet or fructose-containing drink water [22, 23, 26, 36, 125-127]. To recapitulate these findings, Le et al. [128] conducted a controlled clinical trial to assess the effects of fructose on ectopic fat accumulation. They report that a seven-day high-fructose diet is sufficient to cause abnormal lipid deposition in the liver of healthy subjects. Furthermore, they show that subjects with a family history of type 2 diabetes are more prone to developing dyslipidemia with concomitant onset of NAFLD, when challenged persistently by high fructose intake. Likewise, Ouyang et al. [129] report that consumption of fructose in patients with NAFLD is nearly 2- to 3-fold higher than gender- and BMI-matched controls subjects. Consistent with these observations, a 2-fold induction of ketohexokinase (KHK), a key hepatic enzyme in fructose catabolism, is detected in the liver biopsies of those patients compared to control subjects [129]. A recent study show that increased fructose consumption is associated with fibrosis severity in patients with NALFD [130]. Together these data are consistent with the idea that high fructose consumption may play a causative role in the development of NAFLD.

Mechanistic Insight into Fructose-Induced Fatty Liver Disease

It is known that fructose is mainly metabolized in the liver [9]. Increased fructose influx into the liver promotes de novo lipogenesis, culminating in the induction of sterol regulatory element binding protein 1c (SREBP-1c), a master regulator of the lipogenic pathway in the liver [22, 131, 132]. Augmented SREBP-1 activity stimulates the production of fatty acid synthase (FAS) and acetyl coA carboxylase (ACC), favoring fat accumulation in the liver [131, 132]. Interestingly, glucose and fructose exerts different effects on SREBP-1c expression. For example, glucose-rich diets are associated with a transient induction of SREBP-1c expression, whereas high fructose feeding results in extended duration of SREBP-1 production. An underlying interpretation of these data is that fructose, as opposed to glucose, stimulates SREBP-1c-dependent lipogenesis independently of insulin action [133].

In addition to its stimulatory effect on hepatic SREBP-1c activity, high fructose feeding is shown to enhance the expression of peroxisome proliferators-activated receptor-γ co-activator (PGC)-1β in the liver [23]. PGC-1β is characterized as a co-activator that is responsible for binding and activating SREBP-1c [134]. A more recent study by Nagai et al. [126] shows that PGC-1β plays an important role in the development of NAFLD in high fructose-fed rats. Selective inhibition of PGC-1β activity by shRNA-mediated gene silencing is shown to reduce fat accumulation in the liver, contributing to the improvement in plasma lipid profiles in high fructose-fed rats [126]. These data characterize PGC-1β as a contributing factor for fructose-induced NAFLD.

There remains an important question: why the liver cannot rid of excessive lipids to avoid steatosis by accelerating VLDL-triglyceride secretion in response to high fructose feeding? A significant clue to this question derives from the study by Ota et al. [135], who show that hepatic VLDL-triglyceride secretion is subject to regulation by endoplasmic reticulum (ER) stress, an adaptive response that is elicited by the accumulation of unfolded or misfolded proteins in the ER lumen. They show that an increased lipid infiltration into the liver induces

ER stress and compromises the VLDL-triglyceride secretory pathway. This effect inhibits hepatic triglyceride secretion and instigates lipid accumulation, contributing to the development of NAFLD [135]. Indeed, hepatic ER stress along with concomitant steatosis is detectable in the liver of high fructose-fed animals [22, 23, 26, 136]. These results implicate that hepatic ER stress plays an important role in retarding VLDL-triglyceride secretion and ensuing fat accumulation in the liver in response to fructose feeding.

Conclusion

This article is intended to review the effect of fructose on metabolism in the body. Preclinical studies and clinical data have unequivocally demonstrated that excessive intake of fructose is deleterious to glucose and lipid metabolism. Due to the distinct mechanism by which fructose is metabolized in the body, fructose consumption tends to suppress satiety and promote hunger, resulting in overeating. This effect in combination with physical inactivity is causative for the development of undue weight gain. Indeed, fructose overconsumption is attributable to the pathogenesis of insulin resistance and fatty liver disease, two interlocking pathological traits in subjects with morbid obesity and/or type 2 diabetes. Furthermore, excessive fructose intake is linked to the development of hypertriglyceridemia, an atherogenic lipid profile that accounts for increased risk of cardiovascular disease. These data support the idea of limiting excessive fructose addition in beverages and merchandized food to counteract the epidemic of obesity in order to avert the risk of cardiovascular disease and type 2 diabetes.

We would like to stress that our goal in this review is not to discourage dietary intake of fructose from fructose-containing fruits and honey. In addition to fructose content, these natural products contain vitamins, fibers and minerals that are highly beneficial for health. Instead, our objective is to provide an unbaised synopsis of the impact of fructose consumption in its refined form on health and disease. Balanced intake of dietary fructose is recommended to stave off the adverse effect of fructose on the body for preventing against the development of obesity and type 2 diabetes.

Acknowlegment

This study was supported in part by American Diabetes Association and National Health Institute grant DK087764.

References

[1] Tiniakos DG, Vos MB, Brunt EM. Nonalcoholic fatty liver disease: pathology and pathogenesis. *Annu. Rev. Pathol.* 2010; 5:145-71.

[2] Bray GA, Nielsen SJ, Popkin BM. Consumption of high-fructose corn syrup in beverages may play a role in the epidemic of obesity. *Am. J. Clin. Nutr.* 2004; 79:537-43.

[3] Ludwig DS, Peterson KE, Gortmaker SL. Relation between consumption of sugar-sweetened drinks and childhood obesity: a prospective, observational analysis. *Lancet* 2001; 357:505-8.
[4] James J, Kerr D. Prevention of childhood obesity by reducing soft drinks. *Int. J. Obes.* (Lond) 2005; 29 Suppl 2:S54-7.
[5] Philippas NG, Lo CW. Childhood obesity: etiology, prevention, and treatment. *Nutr. Clin. Care.* 2005; 8:77-88.
[6] Gibson SA. Associations between energy density and macronutrient composition in the diets of pre-school children: sugars vs. starch. *Int. J. Obes. Relat. Metab. Disord.* 2000; 24:633-8.
[7] White JS. Straight talk about high-fructose corn syrup: what it is and what it ain't. *Am. J. Clin. Nutr.* 2008; 88:1716S-21S.
[8] Duffey KJ, Popkin BM. High-fructose corn syrup: is this what's for dinner? *Am. J. Clin. Nutr.* 2008; 88:1722S-32S.
[9] Tappy L, Le KA. Metabolic effects of fructose and the worldwide increase in obesity. *Physiol. Rev.* 2010; 90:23-46.
[10] Gaby AR. Adverse effects of dietary fructose. *Altern. Med. Rev.* 2005; 10:294-306.
[11] Tappy L, Le KA, Tran C, Paquot N. Fructose and metabolic diseases: new findings, new questions. *Nutrition* 2010; 26:1044-9.
[12] Samuel VT. Fructose induced lipogenesis: from sugar to fat to insulin resistance. *Trends Endocrinol. Metab.* 2011; 22:60-5.
[13] Smith LH, Jr., Ettinger RH, Seligson D. A comparison of the metabolism of fructose and glucose in hepatic disease and diabetes mellitus. *J. Clin. Invest.* 1953; 32:273-82.
[14] Mayes PA. Intermediary metabolism of fructose. *Am. J. Clin. Nutr.* 1993; 58:754S-65S.
[15] Cherrington AD. Banting Lecture 1997. Control of glucose uptake and release by the liver in vivo. *Diabetes* 1999; 48:1198-214.
[16] Bizeau ME, Pagliassotti MJ. Hepatic adaptations to sucrose and fructose. *Metabolism* 2005; 54:1189-201.
[17] Sato Y, Ito T, Udaka N, Kanisawa M, Noguchi Y, Cushman SW, Satoh S. Immunohistochemical localization of facilitated-diffusion glucose transporters in rat pancreatic islets. *Tissue Cell* 1996; 28:637-43.
[18] Schwartz MW, Porte D, Jr. Diabetes, obesity, and the brain. *Science* 2005; 307:375-9.
[19] Schwartz MW, Woods SC, Porte D, Jr., Seeley RJ, Baskin DG. Central nervous system control of food intake. *Nature* 2000; 404:661-71.
[20] Havel PJ. Control of energy homeostasis and insulin action by adipocyte hormones: leptin, acylation stimulating protein, and adiponectin. *Curr. Opin. Lipidol.* 2002; 13:51-9.
[21] Woods SC, Porte D, Jr., Bobbioni E, Ionescu E, Sauter JF, Rohner-Jeanrenaud F, Jeanrenaud B. Insulin: its relationship to the central nervous system and to the control of food intake and body weight. *Am. J. Clin. Nutr.* 1985; 42:1063-71.
[22] Basciano H, Federico L, Adeli K. Fructose, insulin resistance, and metabolic dyslipidemia. *Nutr. Metab.* (Lond) 2005; 2:5.
[23] Qu S, Su D, Altomonte J, Kamagate A, He J, Perdomo G, Tse T, Jiang Y, Dong HH. PPAR{alpha} mediates the hypolipidemic action of fibrates by antagonizing FoxO1. *Am. J. Physiol. Endocrinol. Metab.* 2007; 292:E421-34.

[24] Ebbeling CB, Feldman HA, Osganian SK, Chomitz VR, Ellenbogen SJ, Ludwig DS. Effects of decreasing sugar-sweetened beverage consumption on body weight in adolescents: a randomized, controlled pilot study. *Pediatrics* 2006; 117:673-80.

[25] Havel PJ. Dietary fructose: implications for dysregulation of energy homeostasis and lipid/carbohydrate metabolism. *Nutr. Rev.* 2005; 63:133-57.

[26] Zhang L, Perdomo G, Kim DH, Qu S, Ringquist S, Trucco M, Dong HH. Proteomic analysis of fructose-induced fatty liver in hamsters. *Metabolism* 2008; 57:1115-24.

[27] Grundy SM. Multifactorial causation of obesity: implications for prevention. *Am. J. Clin. Nutr.* 1998; 67:563S-72S.

[28] Montonen J, Jarvinen R, Knekt P, Heliovaara M, Reunanen A. Consumption of sweetened beverages and intakes of fructose and glucose predict type 2 diabetes occurrence. *J. Nutr.* 2007; 137:1447-54.

[29] Hill JO, Wyatt HR, Reed GW, Peters JC. Obesity and the environment: where do we go from here? *Science* 2003; 299:853-5.

[30] Hill JO, Peters JC. Environmental contributions to the obesity epidemic. *Science* 1998; 280:1371-4.

[31] French SA, Story M, Jeffery RW. Environmental influences on eating and physical activity. *Annu. Rev. Public. Health.* 2001; 22:309-35.

[32] Cohen JC, Horton JD, Hobbs HH. Human fatty liver disease: old questions and new insights. *Science* 2011; 332:1519-23.

[33] Friedman JM. A war on obesity, not the obese. *Science* 2003; 299:856-8.

[34] Marriott BP, Cole N, Lee E. National estimates of dietary fructose intake increased from 1977 to 2004 in the United States. *J. Nutr.* 2009; 139:1228S-35S.

[35] Stanhope KL, Schwarz JM, Keim NL, Griffen SC, Bremer AA, Graham JL, Hatcher B, Cox CL, Dyachenko A, Zhang W, McGahan JP, Seibert A, Krauss RM, Chiu S, Schaefer EJ, Ai M, Otokozawa S, Nakajima K, Nakano T, Beysen C, Hellerstein MK, Berglund L, Havel PJ. Consuming fructose-sweetened, not glucose-sweetened, beverages increases visceral adiposity and lipids and decreases insulin sensitivity in overweight/obese humans. *J. Clin. Invest.* 2009; 119:1322-34.

[36] Jurgens H, Haass W, Castaneda TR, Schurmann A, Koebnick C, Dombrowski F, Otto B, Nawrocki AR, Scherer PE, Spranger J, Ristow M, Joost HG, Havel PJ, Tschop MH. Consuming fructose-sweetened beverages increases body adiposity in mice. *Obes. Res.* 2005; 13:1146-56.

[37] Bugianesi E, Zannoni C, Vanni E, Marzocchi R, Marchesini G. Non-alcoholic fatty liver and insulin resistance: a cause-effect relationship? *Dig. Liver. Dis.* 2004; 36:165-73.

[38] Au CS, Wagner A, Chong T, Qiu W, Sparks JD, Adeli K. Insulin regulates hepatic apolipoprotein B production independent of the mass or activity of Akt1/PKBalpha. *Metabolism* 2004; 53:228-35.

[39] Li P, Koike T, Qin B, Kubota M, Kawata Y, Jia YJ, Oshida Y. A high-fructose diet impairs Akt and PKCzeta phosphorylation and GLUT4 translocation in rat skeletal muscle. *Horm. Metab. Res.* 2008; 40:528-32.

[40] Li JM, Li YC, Kong LD, Hu QH. Curcumin inhibits hepatic protein-tyrosine phosphatase 1B and prevents hypertriglyceridemia and hepatic steatosis in fructose-fed rats. *Hepatology* 2010; 51:1555-66.

[41] Bezerra RM, Ueno M, Silva MS, Tavares DQ, Carvalho CR, Saad MJ. A high fructose diet affects the early steps of insulin action in muscle and liver of rats. *J. Nutr.* 2000; 130:1531-5.

[42] Wei Y, Wang D, Pagliassotti MJ. Fructose selectively modulates c-jun N-terminal kinase activity and insulin signaling in rat primary hepatocytes. *J. Nutr.* 2005; 135:1642-6.

[43] Wei Y, Pagliassotti MJ. Hepatospecific effects of fructose on c-jun NH2-terminal kinase: implications for hepatic insulin resistance. *Am. J. Physiol. Endocrinol. Metab.* 2004; 287:E926-33.

[44] Wei Y, Wang D, Topczewski F, Pagliassotti MJ. Fructose-mediated stress signaling in the liver: implications for hepatic insulin resistance. *J. Nutr. Biochem.* 2007; 18:1-9.

[45] Lim JS, Mietus-Snyder M, Valente A, Schwarz JM, Lustig RH. The role of fructose in the pathogenesis of NAFLD and the metabolic syndrome. *Nat. Rev. Gastroenterol. Hepatol.* 2010; 7:251-64.

[46] Zhang Y, Proenca R, Maffei M, Barone M, Leopold L, Friedman JM. Positional cloning of the mouse obese gene and its human homologue. *Nature* 1994; 372:425-32.

[47] Caro JF, Sinha MK, Kolaczynski JW, Zhang PL, Considine RV. Leptin: the tale of an obesity gene. *Diabetes* 1996; 45:1455-62.

[48] Montague CT, Farooqi IS, Whitehead JP, Soos MA, Rau H, Wareham NJ, Sewter CP, Digby JE, Mohammed SN, Hurst JA, Cheetham CH, Earley AR, Barnett AH, Prins JB, O'Rahilly S. Congenital leptin deficiency is associated with severe early-onset obesity in humans. *Nature* 1997; 387:903-8.

[49] Clement K, Vaisse C, Lahlou N, Cabrol S, Pelloux V, Cassuto D, Gourmelen M, Dina C, Chambaz J, Lacorte JM, Basdevant A, Bougneres P, Lebouc Y, Froguel P, Guy-Grand B. A mutation in the human leptin receptor gene causes obesity and pituitary dysfunction. *Nature* 1998; 392:398-401.

[50] Farooqi IS, Jebb SA, Langmack G, Lawrence E, Cheetham CH, Prentice AM, Hughes IA, McCamish MA, O'Rahilly S. Effects of recombinant leptin therapy in a child with congenital leptin deficiency. *N. Engl. J. Med.* 1999; 341:879-84.

[51] Bluher S, Mantzoros CS. Leptin in humans: lessons from translational research. *Am. J. Clin. Nutr.* 2009; 89:991S-7S.

[52] Mulligan K, Khatami H, Schwarz JM, Sakkas GK, DePaoli AM, Tai VW, Wen MJ, Lee GA, Grunfeld C, Schambelan M. The effects of recombinant human leptin on visceral fat, dyslipidemia, and insulin resistance in patients with human immunodeficiency virus-associated lipoatrophy and hypoleptinemia. *J. Clin. Endocrinol. Metab.* 2009; 94:1137-44.

[53] Teff KL, Grudziak J, Townsend RR, Dunn TN, Grant RW, Adams SH, Keim NL, Cummings BP, Stanhope KL, Havel PJ. Endocrine and metabolic effects of consuming fructose- and glucose-sweetened beverages with meals in obese men and women: influence of insulin resistance on plasma triglyceride responses. *J. Clin. Endocrinol. Metab.* 2009; 94:1562-9.

[54] Adams SH, Stanhope KL, Grant RW, Cummings BP, Havel PJ. Metabolic and endocrine profiles in response to systemic infusion of fructose and glucose in rhesus macaques. *Endocrinology* 2008; 149:3002-8.

[55] Mueller WM, Gregoire FM, Stanhope KL, Mobbs CV, Mizuno TM, Warden CH, Stern JS, Havel PJ. Evidence that glucose metabolism regulates leptin secretion from cultured rat adipocytes. *Endocrinology* 1998; 139:551-8.

[56] Havel PJ. Control of energy homeostasis and insulin action by adipocyte hormones: leptin, acylation stimulating protein, and adiponectin. *Curr. Opin. Lipidol.* 2002; 13:51-9.

[57] Elliott SS, Keim NL, Stern JS, Teff K, Havel PJ. Fructose, weight gain, and the insulin resistance syndrome. *Am. J. Clin. Nutr.* 2002; 76:911-22.

[58] Shapiro A, Mu W, Roncal C, Cheng KY, Johnson RJ, Scarpace PJ. Fructose-induced leptin resistance exacerbates weight gain in response to subsequent high-fat feeding. *Am. J. Physiol. Regul. Integr. Comp. Physiol* 2008; 295:R1370-5.

[59] Vila L, Roglans N, Alegret M, Sanchez RM, Vazquez-Carrera M, Laguna JC. Suppressor of cytokine signaling-3 (SOCS-3) and a deficit of serine/threonine (Ser/Thr) phosphoproteins involved in leptin transduction mediate the effect of fructose on rat liver lipid metabolism. *Hepatology* 2008; 48:1506-16.

[60] Teff KL, Elliott SS, Tschop M, Kieffer TJ, Rader D, Heiman M, Townsend RR, Keim NL, D'Alessio D, Havel PJ. Dietary fructose reduces circulating insulin and leptin, attenuates postprandial suppression of ghrelin, and increases triglycerides in women. *J. Clin. Endocrinol. Metab.* 2004; 89:2963-72.

[61] Tschop M, Wawarta R, Riepl RL, Friedrich S, Bidlingmaier M, Landgraf R, Folwaczny C. Post-prandial decrease of circulating human ghrelin levels. *J. Endocrinol. Invest.* 2001; 24:RC19-21.

[62] Wren AM, Small CJ, Ward HL, Murphy KG, Dakin CL, Taheri S, Kennedy AR, Roberts GH, Morgan DG, Ghatei MA, Bloom SR. The novel hypothalamic peptide ghrelin stimulates food intake and growth hormone secretion. *Endocrinology* 2000; 141:4325-8.

[63] Wren AM, Seal LJ, Cohen MA, Brynes AE, Frost GS, Murphy KG, Dhillo WS, Ghatei MA, Bloom SR. Ghrelin enhances appetite and increases food intake in humans. *J. Clin. Endocrinol. Metab.* 2001; 86:5992.

[64] Nakazato M, Murakami N, Date Y, Kojima M, Matsuo H, Kangawa K, Matsukura S. A role for ghrelin in the central regulation of feeding. *Nature* 2001; 409:194-8.

[65] Kojima M, Hosoda H, Date Y, Nakazato M, Matsuo H, Kangawa K. Ghrelin is a growth-hormone-releasing acylated peptide from stomach. *Nature* 1999; 402:656-60.

[66] Dornonville de la Cour C, Bjorkqvist M, Sandvik AK, Bakke I, Zhao CM, Chen D, Hakanson R. A-like cells in the rat stomach contain ghrelin and do not operate under gastrin control. *Regul. Pept.* 2001; 99:141-50.

[67] Date Y, Kojima M, Hosoda H, Sawaguchi A, Mondal MS, Suganuma T, Matsukura S, Kangawa K, Nakazato M. Ghrelin, a novel growth hormone-releasing acylated peptide, is synthesized in a distinct endocrine cell type in the gastrointestinal tracts of rats and humans. *Endocrinology* 2000; 141:4255-61.

[68] Korbonits M, Kojima M, Kangawa K, Grossman AB. Presence of ghrelin in normal and adenomatous human pituitary. *Endocrine* 2001; 14:101-4.

[69] Mori K, Yoshimoto A, Takaya K, Hosoda K, Ariyasu H, Yahata K, Mukoyama M, Sugawara A, Hosoda H, Kojima M, Kangawa K, Nakao K. Kidney produces a novel acylated peptide, ghrelin. *FEBS Lett.* 2000; 486:213-6.

[70] Gualillo O, Caminos J, Blanco M, Garcia-Caballero T, Kojima M, Kangawa K, Dieguez C, Casanueva F. Ghrelin, a novel placental-derived hormone. *Endocrinology* 2001; 142:788-94.

[71] Mondal MS, Date Y, Yamaguchi H, Toshinai K, Tsuruta T, Kangawa K, Nakazato M. Identification of ghrelin and its receptor in neurons of the rat arcuate nucleus. *Regul. Pept.* 2005; 126:55-9.

[72] Kojima M, Hosoda H, Matsuo H, Kangawa K. Ghrelin: discovery of the natural endogenous ligand for the growth hormone secretagogue receptor. *Trends Endocrinol. Metab.* 2001; 12:118-22.

[73] Takaya K, Ariyasu H, Kanamoto N, Iwakura H, Yoshimoto A, Harada M, Mori K, Komatsu Y, Usui T, Shimatsu A, Ogawa Y, Hosoda K, Akamizu T, Kojima M, Kangawa K, Nakao K. Ghrelin strongly stimulates growth hormone release in humans. *J. Clin. Endocrinol. Metab.* 2000; 85:4908-11.

[74] Date Y, Murakami N, Kojima M, Kuroiwa T, Matsukura S, Kangawa K, Nakazato M. Central effects of a novel acylated peptide, ghrelin, on growth hormone release in rats. *Biochem. Biophys. Res. Commun.* 2000; 275:477-80.

[75] Seoane LM, Tovar S, Baldelli R, Arvat E, Ghigo E, Casanueva FF, Dieguez C. Ghrelin elicits a marked stimulatory effect on GH secretion in freely-moving rats. *Eur. J. Endocrinol.* 2000; 143:R7-9.

[76] Tolle V, Zizzari P, Tomasetto C, Rio MC, Epelbaum J, Bluet-Pajot MT. In vivo and in vitro effects of ghrelin/motilin-related peptide on growth hormone secretion in the rat. *Neuroendocrinology* 2001; 73:54-61.

[77] Kamegai J, Tamura H, Shimizu T, Ishii S, Sugihara H, Wakabayashi I. Central effect of ghrelin, an endogenous growth hormone secretagogue, on hypothalamic peptide gene expression. *Endocrinology* 2000; 141:4797-800.

[78] Tschop M, Smiley DL, Heiman ML. Ghrelin induces adiposity in rodents. *Nature* 2000; 407:908-13.

[79] Asakawa A, Inui A, Kaga T, Yuzuriha H, Nagata T, Ueno N, Makino S, Fujimiya M, Niijima A, Fujino MA, Kasuga M. Ghrelin is an appetite-stimulatory signal from stomach with structural resemblance to motilin. *Gastroenterology* 2001; 120:337-45.

[80] Nakagawa T, Hu H, Zharikov S, Tuttle KR, Short RA, Glushakova O, Ouyang X, Feig DI, Block ER, Herrera-Acosta J, Patel JM, Johnson RJ. A causal role for uric acid in fructose-induced metabolic syndrome. *Am. J. Physiol. Renal. Physiol.* 2006; 290:F625-31.

[81] Shintani M, Ogawa Y, Ebihara K, Aizawa-Abe M, Miyanaga F, Takaya K, Hayashi T, Inoue G, Hosoda K, Kojima M, Kangawa K, Nakao K. Ghrelin, an endogenous growth hormone secretagogue, is a novel orexigenic peptide that antagonizes leptin action through the activation of hypothalamic neuropeptide Y/Y1 receptor pathway. *Diabetes* 2001; 50:227-32.

[82] Arvat E, Di Vito L, Broglio F, Papotti M, Muccioli G, Dieguez C, Casanueva FF, Deghenghi R, Camanni F, Ghigo E. Preliminary evidence that Ghrelin, the natural GH secretagogue (GHS)-receptor ligand, strongly stimulates GH secretion in humans. *J. Endocrinol. Invest.* 2000; 23:493-5.

[83] Broglio F, Arvat E, Benso A, Gottero C, Muccioli G, Papotti M, van der Lely AJ, Deghenghi R, Ghigo E. Ghrelin, a natural GH secretagogue produced by the stomach, induces hyperglycemia and reduces insulin secretion in humans. *J. Clin. Endocrinol. Metab.* 2001; 86:5083-6.

[84] Horvath TL, Diano S, Sotonyi P, Heiman M, Tschop M. Minireview: ghrelin and the regulation of energy balance--a hypothalamic perspective. *Endocrinology* 2001; 142:4163-9.

[85] Tschop M, Weyer C, Tataranni PA, Devanarayan V, Ravussin E, Heiman ML. Circulating ghrelin levels are decreased in human obesity. *Diabetes* 2001; 50:707-9.

[86] Lindqvist A, Baelemans A, Erlanson-Albertsson C. Effects of sucrose, glucose and fructose on peripheral and central appetite signals. *Regul. Pept.* 2008; 150:26-32.

[87] Spruss A, Kanuri G, Wagnerberger S, Haub S, Bischoff SC, Bergheim I. Toll-like receptor 4 is involved in the development of fructose-induced hepatic steatosis in mice. *Hepatology* 2009; 50:1094-104.

[88] Tsai J, Zhang R, Qiu W, Su Q, Naples M, Adeli K. Inflammatory NF-kappaB activation promotes hepatic apolipoprotein B100 secretion: evidence for a link between hepatic inflammation and lipoprotein production. *Am. J. Physiol. Gastrointest. Liver Physiol.* 2009; 296:G1287-98.

[89] Haub S, Kanuri G, Volynets V, Brune T, Bischoff SC, Bergheim I. Serotonin reuptake transporter (SERT) plays a critical role in the onset of fructose-induced hepatic steatosis in mice. *Am. J. Physiol. Gastrointest. Liver Physiol.* 2010; 298:G335-44.

[90] Tetri LH, Basaranoglu M, Brunt EM, Yerian LM, Neuschwander-Tetri BA. Severe NAFLD with hepatic necroinflammatory changes in mice fed trans fats and a high-fructose corn syrup equivalent. *Am. J. Physiol. Gastrointest. Liver Physiol.* 2008; 295:G987-95.

[91] Sanchez-Lozada LG, Mu W, Roncal C, Sautin YY, Abdelmalek M, Reungjui S, Le M, Nakagawa T, Lan HY, Yu X, Johnson RJ. Comparison of free fructose and glucose to sucrose in the ability to cause fatty liver. *Eur. J. Nutr.* 2010; 49:1-9.

[92] Roglans N, Vila L, Farre M, Alegret M, Sanchez RM, Vazquez-Carrera M, Laguna JC. Impairment of hepatic Stat-3 activation and reduction of PPARalpha activity in fructose-fed rats. *Hepatology* 2007; 45:778-88.

[93] Qin B, Anderson RA, Adeli K. Tumor necrosis factor-alpha directly stimulates the overproduction of hepatic apolipoprotein B100-containing VLDL via impairment of hepatic insulin signaling. *Am. J. Physiol. Gastrointest. Liver Physiol.* 2008; 294:G1120-9.

[94] Qin B, Qiu W, Avramoglu RK, Adeli K. Tumor necrosis factor-alpha induces intestinal insulin resistance and stimulates the overproduction of intestinal apolipoprotein B48-containing lipoproteins. *Diabetes* 2007; 56:450-61.

[95] Kanuri G, Spruss A, Wagnerberger S, Bischoff SC, Bergheim I. Role of tumor necrosis factor alpha (TNFalpha) in the onset of fructose-induced nonalcoholic fatty liver disease in mice. *J. Nutr. Biochem.* 2011; 22:527-34.

[96] Murphy SP, Johnson RK. The scientific basis of recent US guidance on sugars intake. *Am. J. Clin. Nutr.* 2003; 78:827S-33S.

[97] Martinez FJ, Rizza RA, Romero JC. High-fructose feeding elicits insulin resistance, hyperinsulinism, and hypertension in normal mongrel dogs. *Hypertension* 1994; 23:456-63.

[98] Hwang IS, Ho H, Hoffman BB, Reaven GM. Fructose-induced insulin resistance and hypertension in rats. *Hypertension* 1987; 10:512-6.

[99] Kohen-Avramoglu R, Theriault A, Adeli K. Emergence of the metabolic syndrome in childhood: an epidemiological overview and mechanistic link to dyslipidemia. *Clin. Biochem.* 2003; 36:413-20.

[100] Brown CM, Dulloo AG, Yepuri G, Montani JP. Fructose ingestion acutely elevates blood pressure in healthy young humans. *Am. J. Physiol. Regul. Integr. Comp. Physiol.* 2008; 294:R730-7.

[101] Brown CM, Dulloo AG, Montani JP. Sugary drinks in the pathogenesis of obesity and cardiovascular diseases. *Int. J. Obes.* (Lond) 2008; 32 Suppl 6:S28-34.

[102] Kelley GL, Allan G, Azhar S. High dietary fructose induces a hepatic stress response resulting in cholesterol and lipid dysregulation. *Endocrinology* 2004; 145:548-55.

[103] Ginsberg HN. Treatment for patients with the metabolic syndrome. *Am. J. Cardiol.* 2003; 91:29E-39E.

[104] Moller DE, Kaufman KD. Metabolic syndrome: a clinical and molecular perspective. *Annu. Rev. Med.* 2005; 56:45-62.

[105] Ostos MA, Recalde D, Baroukh N, Callejo A, Rouis M, Castro G, Zakin MM. Fructose intake increases hyperlipidemia and modifies apolipoprotein expression in apolipoprotein AI-CIII-AIV transgenic mice. *J. Nutr.* 2002; 132:918-23.

[106] Taghibiglou C, Carpentier A, Van Iderstine SC, Chen B, Rudy D, Aiton A, Lewis GF, Adeli K. Mechanisms of hepatic very low density lipoprotein overproduction in insulin resistance. Evidence for enhanced lipoprotein assembly, reduced intracellular ApoB degradation, and increased microsomal triglyceride transfer protein in a fructose-fed hamster model. *J. Biol. Chem.* 2000; 275:8416-25.

[107] Kasim-Karakas SE, Vriend H, Almario R, Chow LC, Goodman MN. Effects of dietary carbohydrates on glucose and lipid metabolism in golden Syrian hamsters. *J. Lab. Clin. Med.* 1996; 128:208-13.

[108] Taghibiglou C, Rashid-Kolvear F, Van Iderstine SC, Le-Tien H, Fantus IG, Lewis GF, Adeli K. Hepatic very low density lipoprotein-ApoB overproduction is associated with attenuated hepatic insulin signaling and overexpression of protein-tyrosine phosphatase 1B in a fructose-fed hamster model of insulin resistance. *J. Biol. Chem.* 2002; 277:793-803.

[109] Kamagate A, Qu S, Perdomo G, Su D, Kim DH, Slusher S, Meseck M, Dong HH. FoxO1 mediates insulin-dependent regulation of hepatic VLDL production in mice. *J. Clin. Invest.* 2008; 118:2347-64.

[110] Kamagate A, Dong HH. FoxO1 integrates insulin signaling to VLDL production. *Cell Cycle* 2008; 7:3162-70.

[111] Haidari M, Leung N, Mahbub F, Uffelman KD, Kohen-Avramoglu R, Lewis GF, Adeli K. Fasting and postprandial overproduction of intestinally derived lipoproteins in an animal model of insulin resistance. Evidence that chronic fructose feeding in the hamster is accompanied by enhanced intestinal de novo lipogenesis and ApoB48-containing lipoprotein overproduction. *J. Biol. Chem.* 2002; 277:31646-55.

[112] Brodsky JL, Fisher EA. The many intersecting pathways underlying apolipoprotein B secretion and degradation. *Trends Endocrinol. Metab.* 2008; 19:254-9.

[113] Tanoli T, Yue P, Yablonskiy D, Schonfeld G. Fatty liver in familial hypobetalipoproteinemia: roles of the APOB defects, intra-abdominal adipose tissue, and insulin sensitivity. *J. Lipid. Res.* 2004; 45:941-7.

[114] Tietge UJ, Bakillah A, Maugeais C, Tsukamoto K, Hussain M, Rader DJ. Hepatic overexpression of microsomal triglyceride transfer protein (MTP) results in increased in vivo secretion of VLDL triglycerides and apolipoprotein B. *J. Lipid. Res.* 1999; 40:2134-9.

[115] Jamil H, Chu CH, Dickson JK, Jr., Chen Y, Yan M, Biller SA, Gregg RE, Wetterau JR, Gordon DA. Evidence that microsomal triglyceride transfer protein is limiting in the production of apolipoprotein B-containing lipoproteins in hepatic cells. *J. Lipid. Res.* 1998; 39:1448-54.

[116] Hussain MM, Shi J, Dreizen P. Microsomal triglyceride transfer protein and its role in apoB-lipoprotein assembly. *J. Lipid. Res.* 2003; 44:22-32.

[117] Wang C, McConathy WJ, Kloer HJ, Alaupovic P. Modulation of lipoprotein lipase activity by apolipoproteins: effect of apolipoprotein C-III. *J. Clin. Invest.* 1985; 75:384.

[118] McConathy WJ, Gesquiere JC, Bass H, Tartar A, Fruchart JC. Inhibition of lipoprotein lipase activity by synthetic peptides of apolipoprotein C-III. *J. Lipid. Res.* 1992; 33:995-1003.

[119] Kinnunen PKJ, Ehnholm C. Effect of serum and C apolipoproteins from very low density lipoproteins on human post-heparin plasma hepatic lipase. *FEBS Lett.* 1976; 65:354-7.

[120] Altomonte J, Cong L, Harbaran S, Richter A, Xu J, Meseck M, Dong HH. Foxo1 Mediates Insulin Action on ApoC-III and Triglyceride Metabolism. *J. Clin. Invest.* 2004; 114:1493-503.

[121] Carpentier A, Taghibiglou C, Leung N, Szeto L, Van Iderstine SC, Uffelman KD, Buckingham R, Adeli K, Lewis GF. Ameliorated hepatic insulin resistance is associated with normalization of microsomal triglyceride transfer protein expression and reduction in very low density lipoprotein assembly and secretion in the fructose-fed hamster. *J. Biol. Chem.* 2002; 277:28795-802.

[122] Avramoglu RK, Qiu W, Adeli K. Mechanisms of metabolic dyslipidemia in insulin resistant states: deregulation of hepatic and intestinal lipoprotein secretion. *Front. Biosci.* 2003; 8:d464-76.

[123] Nakae J, Barr V, Accili D. Differential regulation of gene expression by insulin and IGF-1 receptors correlates with phosphorylation of a single amino acid residue in the forkhead transcription factor FKHR. *EMBO J.* 2000; 19:989-96.

[124] Browning JD, Szczepaniak LS, Dobbins R, Nuremberg P, Horton JD, Cohen JC, Grundy SM, Hobbs HH. Prevalence of hepatic steatosis in an urban population in the United States: impact of ethnicity. *Hepatology* 2004; 40:1387-95.

[125] Collison KS, Saleh SM, Bakheet RH, Al-Rabiah RK, Inglis AL, Makhoul NJ, Maqbool ZM, Zaidi MZ, Al-Johi MA, Al-Mohanna FA. Diabetes of the Liver: *The Link Between Nonalcoholic Fatty Liver Disease and HFCS-55*. Obesity (Silver Spring) 2009.

[126] Nagai Y, Yonemitsu S, Erion DM, Iwasaki T, Stark R, Weismann D, Dong J, Zhang D, Jurczak MJ, Loffler MG, Cresswell J, Yu XX, Murray SF, Bhanot S, Monia BP, Bogan JS, Samuel V, Shulman GI. The role of peroxisome proliferator-activated receptor gamma coactivator-1 beta in the pathogenesis of fructose-induced insulin resistance. *Cell Metab.* 2009; 9:252-64.

[127] Ackerman Z, Oron-Herman M, Grozovski M, Rosenthal T, Pappo O, Link G, Sela BA. Fructose-induced fatty liver disease: hepatic effects of blood pressure and plasma triglyceride reduction. *Hypertension* 2005; 45:1012-8.

[128] Le KA, Ith M, Kreis R, Faeh D, Bortolotti M, Tran C, Boesch C, Tappy L. Fructose overconsumption causes dyslipidemia and ectopic lipid deposition in healthy subjects with and without a family history of type 2 diabetes. *Am. J. Clin. Nutr.* 2009; 89:1760-5.

[129] Ouyang X, Cirillo P, Sautin Y, McCall S, Bruchette JL, Diehl AM, Johnson RJ, Abdelmalek MF. Fructose consumption as a risk factor for non-alcoholic fatty liver disease. *J. Hepatol.* 2008; 48:993-9.

[130] Abdelmalek MF, Suzuki A, Guy C, Unalp-Arida A, Colvin R, Johnson RJ, Diehl AM. Increased fructose consumption is associated with fibrosis severity in patients with nonalcoholic fatty liver disease. *Hepatology* 2010; 51:1961-71.

[131] Foretz M, Guichard C, Ferre P, Foufelle F. Sterol regulatory element binding protein-1c is a major mediator of insulin action on the hepatic expression of glucokinase and lipogenesis-related genes. *Proc. Natl. Acad. Sci. USA* 1999; 96:12737-42.

[132] Foretz M, Pacot C, Dugail I, Lemarchand P, Guichard C, Le Liepvre X, Berthelier-Lubrano C, Spiegelman B, Kim JB, Ferre P, Foufelle F. ADD1/SREBP-1c is required in the activation of hepatic lipogenic gene expression by glucose. *Mol. Cell Biol.* 1999; 19:3760-8.

[133] Winder WW, Holmes BF, Rubink DS, Jensen EB, Chen M, Holloszy JO. Activation of AMP-activated protein kinase increases mitochondrial enzymes in skeletal muscle. *J. Appl. Physiol.* 2000; 88:2219-26.

[134] Lin J, Yang R, Tarr PT, Wu PH, Handschin C, Li S, Yang W, Pei L, Uldry M, Tontonoz P, Newgard CB, Spiegelman BM. Hyperlipidemic effects of dietary saturated fats mediated through PGC-1beta coactivation of SREBP. *Cell* 2005; 120:261-73.

[135] Ota T, Gayet C, Ginsberg HN. Inhibition of apolipoprotein B100 secretion by lipid-induced hepatic endoplasmic reticulum stress in rodents. *J. Clin. Invest.* 2008; 118:316-32.

[136] Morand JP, Macri J, Adeli K. Proteomic profiling of hepatic endoplasmic reticulum-associated proteins in an animal model of insulin resistance and metabolic dyslipidemia. *J. Biol. Chem.* 2005; 280:17626-33.

In: Fructose
Editors: Brandon M. Johnston and Aaron B. Collins
ISBN: 978-1-62081-126-9

Chapter 4

DETRIMENTAL EFFECTS OF EXCESSIVE FRUCTOSE INGESTION ON MEMORY AND OTHER BRAIN FUNCTIONS

E. C. Bruggeman[1], A. P. Ross[1], and M. B. Parent[1,2]
[1]Neuroscience Institute, Georgia State University,
Atlanta, Georgia, US
[2]Psychology Department, Georgia State University,
Atlanta, Georgia, US

ABSTRACT

Fructose is a monosaccharide found naturally in fruits, honey, and some vegetables. It also is added to foods in the form of sucrose, concentrated fruit juices, corn syrup, high fructose corn syrup, and crystalline fructose. The addition of fructose to a wide variety of foods and beverages has led to a significant increase in fructose consumption over the past three decades. This is a cause for concern, because excessive intake of fructose causes a variety of pathological effects, including hypertriglyceridemia, visceral adiposity, hyperinsulinemia, non-alcoholic fatty liver disease (NAFLD), elevated inflame-matory factors, insulin resistance, Type 2 diabetes, and hypertension/ cardio-vascular disease. These physiological effects of a high fructose diet are well-documented; in contrast, relatively little is known about the effects of excessive fructose consumption on the central nervous system. The purpose of this chapter is to review the effects of high fructose intake in rodents on the brain, with a particular focus on plasticity and memory. Evidence implicating elevated triglyceride levels, NAFLD, neuroinflammation, and oxidative stress in the pathological effects of a high fructose diet on brain function is presented. Sex-dependent effects of elevated fructose consumption and application of results from experimental models of fructose consumption to the human population also are discussed.

Introduction

Fructose is a monosaccharide found naturally in fruits, honey, and some vegetables. It also is added to foods in the form of sucrose (50% fructose), corn syrup, high fructose corn syrup (42 or 55% fructose), fruit juice concentrates (over 60% of calories in apple juice), and crystalline fructose (almost 100% fructose) [1]. In its various forms, fructose is added to countless foods, including carbonated beverages, fruit products (juices, jams, jellies, and canned fruit), baked goods, cereals, and dairy products [1]. Indeed, it is a challenge for the North American consumer to purchase processed foods that do not contain some form of added fructose.

The addition of fructose to such a wide variety of foods and beverages has led to a significant increase in fructose consumption [2, 3]. Between 1970 and 2005, the average annual intake of high fructose corn syrup increased in the United States from 0.5 pounds to 59 pounds, and the average intake of total sugars increased by 19% [4]. The average American's current fructose intake is estimated to be 10% of total daily energy and is over 17% in the 90th percentile [2]. Overall, men tend to consume more fructose than women, and adolescent boys are the highest consumers, ingesting an average of 75 grams of fructose per day [3]. When body weight is corrected for, however, children 1-10 years of age are the highest consumers, primarily due to consumption of fruits and fruit products [3]. The majority of fructose consumed by the other demographic groups is mostly from added sources [2], rather than from naturally-occurring sources, such as fruit. High fructose corn syrup is largely responsible for the increase in fructose consumption [5-7].

Fructose is metabolized differently than glucose, the other main dietary monosaccharide. Whereas glucose can be metabolized by all cells, fructose is metabolized primarily by the liver [8]. Upon ingestion, fructose is absorbed through the gastrointestinal tract via the GLUT5 transporter [9]. It is then transported to the liver via the hepatic portal vein and subsequently undergoes glycolysis within hepatocytes [8, 10, 11]. An important difference between glucose and fructose metabolism is that fructose metabolism is not regulated by the enzyme phosphofructokinase, which limits the production of triglycerides from glycolysis [11]. By bypassing this rate-limiting step, fructose ingestion results in larger elevations in plasma triglyceride concentrations than does glucose ingestion [12, 13]. Fructose-induced increases in plasma triglyceride concentrations are significant within 3 days [13] and persist as long as high fructose ingestion continues [13, 14]. Another key difference between fructose and glucose is that fructose does not stimulate the release of insulin from the pancreas [15, 16].

Peripheral Effects

When consumed in excessive amounts, a high fructose diet produces large increases in plasma triglyceride concentrations, liver mass [12, 17-20], liver lipid content [19, 21], and visceral adipose tissue [22-24]. Despite these increases, fructose consumption does not typically increase body mass [18, 19, 25], but see [26]. Excess fructose consumption can lead to numerous pathologies in both rodents and humans, including glucose intolerance [27, 28], insulin resistance [29-33], Type 2 diabetes [34, 35], non-alcoholic fatty liver disease

(NAFLD) [36, 37], hypertension [30, 33, 38], oxidative stress [35, 39], and cardiovascular disease [27, 40, 41].

Central Effects

In contrast to the wealth of studies investigating the peripheral consequences of elevated fructose consumption, relatively few studies have focused on the effects of fructose on the central nervous system. One of the first studies to investigate the effects of excessive fructose consumption on brain function tested the effects of feeding hamsters pellets containing 60% fructose for 6 weeks [42]. Brain slices were maintained *ex vivo*, stimulated with insulin, and then several proteins in the insulin signaling cascade were quantified using Western blots. The results indicated that the high fructose diet produced central insulin resistance. Specifically, it reduced phosphorylation of the insulin receptor-β subunit (IR-β), which is the initial step that occurs when insulin binds to the insulin receptor (Figure 1). In addition, the high fructose diet significantly reduced phosphorylation of insulin receptor substrate-1 (IRS-1) and Akt/Protein kinase B (Akt/PKB), two downstream effector proteins in the insulin signaling cascade (Figures 1, 2). In the hippocampus, the high fructose diet decreased protein tyrosine phosphatase, an enzyme involved in regulating the phosphorylation of the insulin signaling proteins, and impaired insulin-induced long-term depression (LTD), a measure of synaptic plasticity.

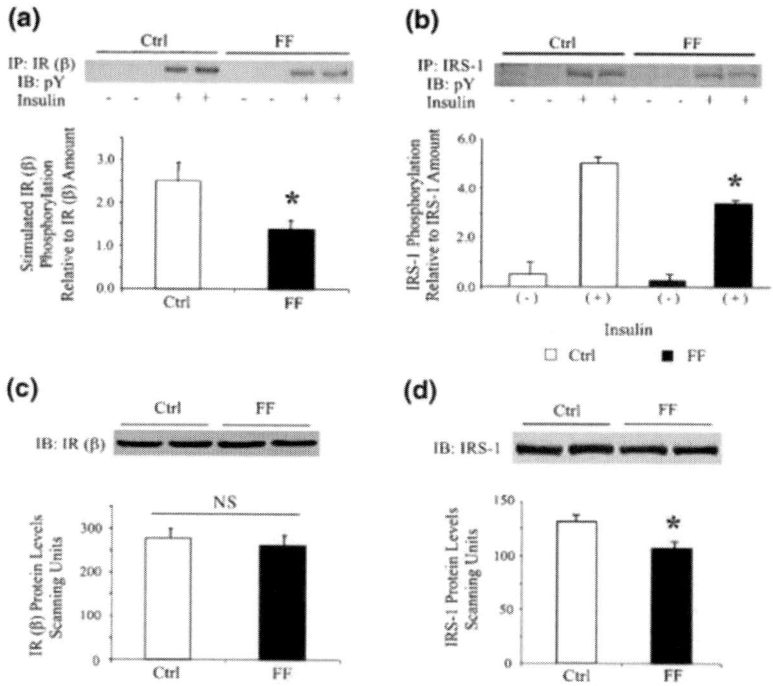

Figure 1. The effects of eating a control (Ctrl) or high fructose diet (60%; FF) on (a) insulin-mediated tyrosine phosphorylation of neural IR-β subunit, (b) insulin-mediated tyrosine phosphorylation of the substrate protein IRS-1, (c) total IR-β protein, and (d) total IRS-1 protein (*$p < 0.05$ vs. control hamsters). From [42] used with permission.

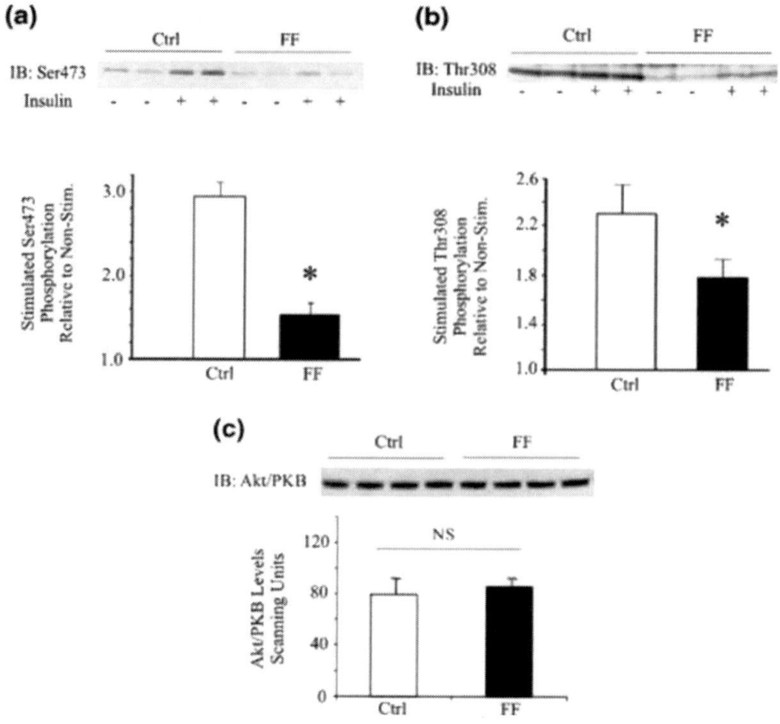

Figure 2. The effects of eating a control (Ctrl) or high fructose diet (60%; FF) on (a) insulin-mediated serine phosphorylation of Akt/PKB protein, (b) insulin-mediated threonine phosphorylation of Akt/PKB protein, and (c) total Akt/PKB protein (*$p < 0.05$ vs. control hamsters). From [42] used with permission.

Since then several other studies have been published indicating that elevated fructose consumption impairs normal brain function in a variety of ways. Rats that are fed a 60% fructose diet for 6 months demonstrate central leptin resistance as indicated by reduced basal phosphorylation levels of signal transducer and activator of transcription 3 (STAT3; a key protein in the leptin signaling cascade) in the hypothalamus [43]. Elevated fructose consumption also produces neuroinflammation. When rats are provided 10% fructose in the drinking water for 4 months, nuclear factor kappa B (NFκB) becomes activated in the cerebral cortex [44]. NF-κB is responsible for initiating the transcription of many different inflammatory factors, and the activation of this protein is a strong indicator of neuro-inflammation [45, 46]. Interleukin-1β and tumor necrosis factor-α, two primary inflammatory factors, also are significantly elevated in the cortices of fructose-drinking rats, as are levels of NADPH oxidase, which indicates oxidative stress [44]. Rats that are given a 23% fructose solution in their drinking water for 1 month have reduced neurogenesis in the dentate gyrus region of the hippocampus [47]. Finally, rats that are given a 10% fructose solution exhibit increased amyloid-β deposits in the cortex and hippocampus [48].

The fact that a high fructose diet disrupts the effects of insulin in hippocampal neurons led us to hypothesize that a high fructose diet would impair memory. This hypothesis is based on the fact that the hippocampus plays a pivotal role in memory [49] and converging lines of evidence indicate that neural insulin signaling facilitates hippocampal-dependent memory [50]. For instance, extensive evidence suggests that peripheral insulin resistance and Type 2 diabetes are associated with deficits in hippocampal-dependent declarative memory [51-55].

In addition, learning and memory of a spatial water maze experience are correlated with activation of the hippocampal insulin signaling pathway [55, 56]. Most importantly, direct infusions of insulin into the hippocampus enhance performance in a variety of memory tasks, and the memory-enhancing effects of hippocampal insulin administration are not observed in diabetic rats [57-59]. Moreover, direct infusion of an insulin antibody into the hippocampus, which blocks insulin signaling, impairs memory [57].

To test whether a high fructose diet would impair memory, we fed adult male rats either a control or 60% fructose diet for 19 weeks and then trained and tested them in the spatial water maze [18]. This is a commonly used behavioral measure of hippocampal function because hippocampal lesions impair memory in this task [60, 61]. Rats were trained to find a submerged platform using extra-maze cues. Learning was assessed by measuring the latency to swim to the platform across training trials. Memory was tested 48 h after training, with the platform absent. Memory measures included 1) time spent in the area of the pool where the platform was previously located (target quadrant), 2) latency to cross the platform location (target), and 3) number of target approaches. Swim speed also was measured to assess behavior not dependent on mnemonic performance.

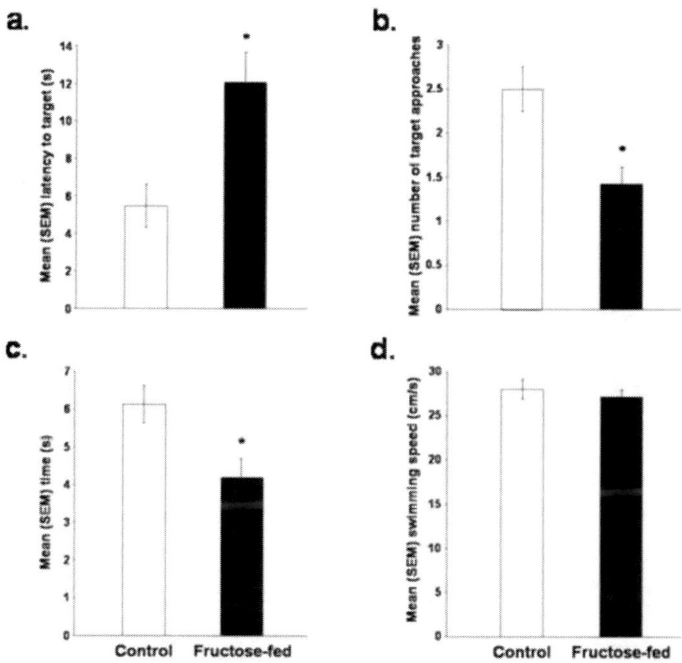

Figure 3. The effects of eating a control or high fructose (60%) diet for 138 days on the mean (+/-) SEM **(a)** latency to reach the target, **(b)** number of target approaches, **(c)** amount of time spent in the target quadrant and **(d)** swim speed during the spatial water maze retention test (*$p < 0.05$ vs. control rats). From [18] used with permission.

The results showed that the high fructose diet impaired memory. Fructose-fed rats exhibited decreased time spent in the target quadrant, an increased latency to reach the target, and fewer number of target approaches (Figures 3A-C). The diet did not impair acquisition performance during training (Figure 4), which suggests that the fructose diet did not influence navigational ability and that the rats were able to learn and retain the location of the platform for short periods of time. The finding that the diet did not affect swim speed supports this interpretation (Figure 3D). Deficits were observed exclusively on the retention test given 48 h after training, which indicates that the diet specifically impaired long-term storage and/or retrieval. Given that postweaning human babies and adolescent males are the highest consumers of fructose [3], we conducted a subsequent study where we fed male rats a 60% fructose diet starting at weaning (postnatal day 21) and continuing into adulthood [62]. As in rats fed the diet starting in adulthood, rats fed the diet at weaning displayed hippocampal-dependent deficits in adulthood.

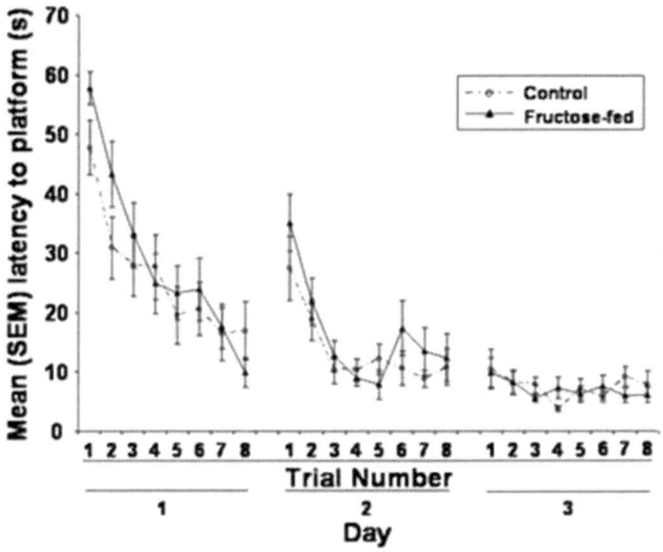

Figure 4. The effects of eating a control or high fructose (60%) diet for 138 days on the mean (+/-) SEM latency to reach the platform during spatial water maze training. From [18] used with permission.

Ingesting excessive amounts of fructose for extensive periods of time does not always impair brain function or memory. For instance, feeding rats a 58% or 60% fructose diet protects them against ischemia reperfusion injury [63, 64]. In addition, elevated fructose consumption enhances learning of a bar-pressing task in mice [65]. We also have observed that female rats may be protected from the effects of a high fructose diet on cognitive function. In another study, we fed female rats a 60% fructose diet starting at weaning for a short (47 d), middle (88 d), or long (144 d) duration [66]. The short and middle durations were selected to test for possible developmental differences, and the long duration was selected because a high fructose diet impairs memory in male rats after 138 days [18]. After their respective diet durations, the rats were tested on an amphetamine self-administration task to test whether a high fructose diet impairs learning that occurs through drug reinforcement. The high fructose diet did not affect rates of acquisition of amphetamine self-administration, the number of infusions earned on either fixed-ratio or progressive-ratio schedules of reinforcement, nor the number of active lever presses during extinction/reinstatement sessions. Follow-up experiments indicated that the 60% fructose diet also did not impair spatial water maze memory in these female rats nor in amphetamine-naïve female rats.

POSSIBLE MECHANISMS

It is likely that fructose acts through multiple processes to produce brain dysfunction, as summarized in Figure 5. As the evidence below will show, fructose could impair brain function by acting directly on brain cells and/or indirectly via one of its metabolic products.

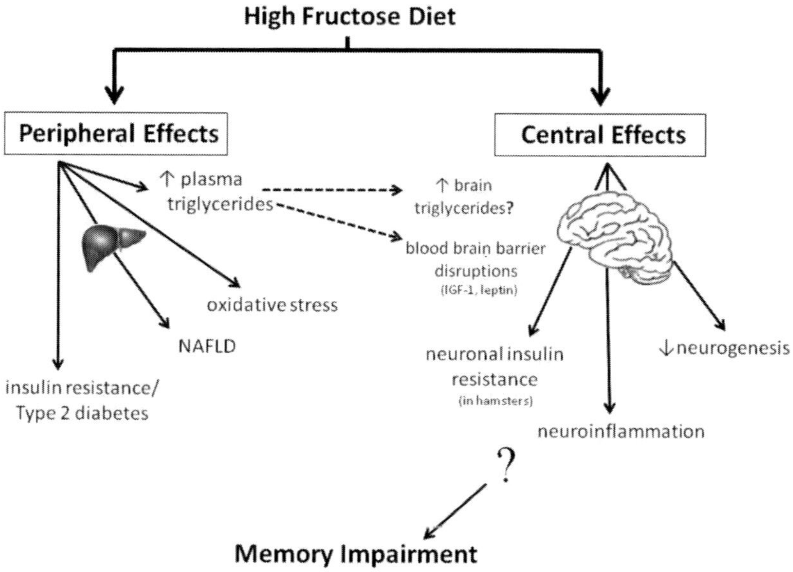

Figure 5. Possible mechanisms through which a high fructose diet may impair memory.

Whether peripheral increases in fructose can have a direct effect on brain function remains to be determined. Several older studies suggest that the transport of fructose across the blood brain barrier is extremely limited [67-69]. Recent evidence, however, suggests that the brain is responsive to fructose. For instance, cerebellar neurons are able to metabolize fructose [70], and fructose sensitive glucose transporters (GLUT5) are found on hippocampal and cortical microglia in both humans and rodents [71]. Importantly, drinking a 20% fructose solution increases expression of GLUT5 in the hippocampus [72]. A recent fMRI human study demonstrated that intravenous fructose infusions decrease cortical activity, whereas glucose infusions increase activity in the same brain regions [73].

Several lines of evidence support the hypothesis that elevated plasma triglyceride concentrations are involved in the memory-impairing effects of a high fructose diet. For instance, high fat diets impair hippocampal-dependent memory [74-76], and pharmacological manipulations that lower plasma triglyceride concentrations reverse the memory-impairing effects of a high fat diet [75]. We have found that the memory-impairing effects of a high fructose diet are slightly, but significantly correlated with the effects of the diet on postmortem plasma triglyceride concentrations (Figures 6A, B), but not with the effects of the diet on plasma free fatty acids, glucose, insulin, or leptin levels (Figures 7A-F) [18]. It also is worth noting that fructose-induced elevations in plasma triglyceride concentrations are less robust in females than in males [66, 77, 78], which may explain, in part, why females are resistant to the memory-impairing effects of a high fructose diet.

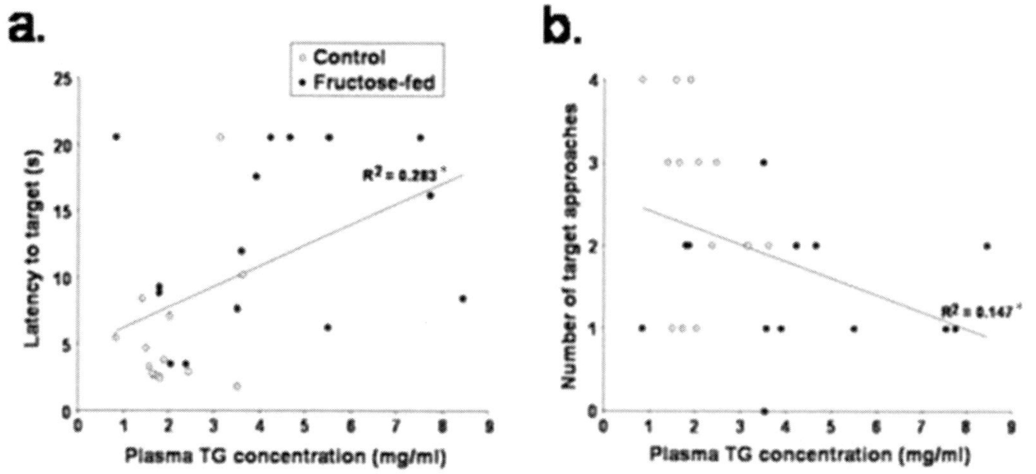

Figure 6. Scatterplots illustrating the association between **(a)** postmortem plasma TG concentrations and latency to reach the target and **(b)** the number of target approaches (*$p < 0.05$ vs. control rats). From [18] used with permission.

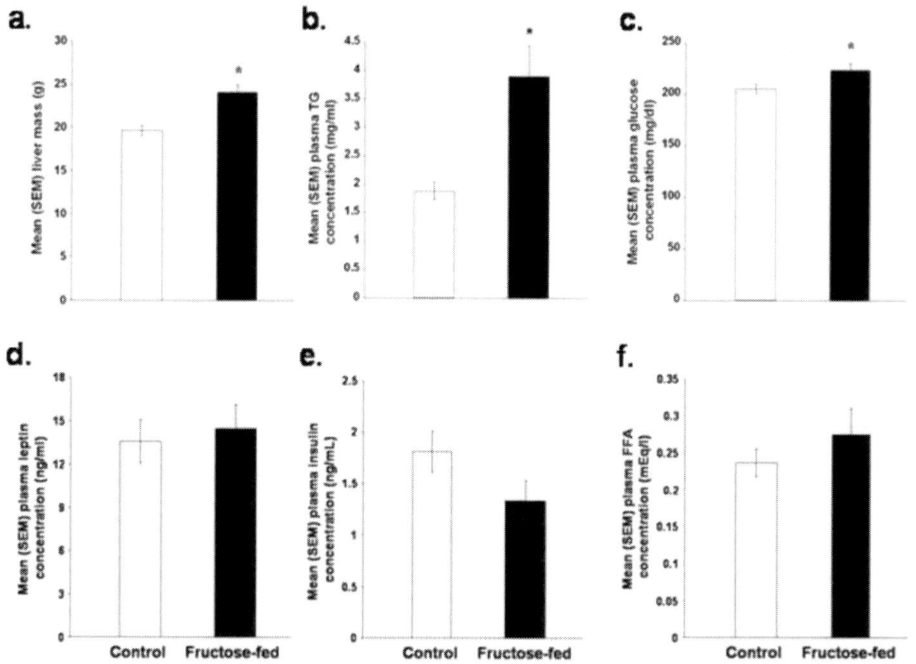

Figure 7. The effects of eating a control or high fructose (60%) diet for 138 days on the mean (+/-) SEM **(a)** liver mass, **(b)** plasma TG concentrations, **(c)** plasma glucose concentrations, **(d)** plasma leptin concentrations, **(e)** plasma insulin concentrations and **(f)** plasma FFA concentrations (*$p < 0.05$ vs. control rats). From [18] used with permission.

Fructose-induced increases in plasma triglyceride concentrations could lead to increases in brain triglyceride concentrations. A high fat diet supplemented with 20% high fructose corn syrup in the drinking water increases cholesterol and disrupts lipid metabolism in the hippocampus [79]. Rats with Type 2 diabetes have significantly higher brain triglyceride concentrations than do control or Type 1 diabetic rats [80]. The involvement of triglycerides in the fructose-induced memory impairment is further supported by evidence showing that direct infusions of the triglyceride triolein into the brain ventricles [81], or the free fatty acid palmitate into the hippocampus [75], impair memory. In addition, application of triolein to hippocampal slices impairs long term potentiation (LTP) [75], the leading candidate synaptic mechanism underlying memory [82].

Fructose-induced elevations in plasma triglyceride concentrations also might impair brain function indirectly, by affecting the transport of substances across the blood brain barrier. For instance, high fat diet-induced elevations in plasma triglyceride concentrations interfere with leptin transport across the blood brain barrier [83]. This is important because peripheral [84] and central [85, 86] administration of leptin enhances memory, including hippocampal-dependent memory. Elevated plasma triglyceride concentrations also prevent insulin-like growth factor (IGF-1) from crossing the blood brain barrier [87]. Peripheral administration of IGF-1 improves memory in diabetic rats [88] and is associated with better cognitive skills in aging humans [89].

Our initial hypothesis was that elevated fructose consumption could impair hippocampal function by producing hippocampal insulin resistance. Although feeding hamsters a 60% fructose diet produces central insulin resistance (Figures 1, 2) [42], research from our laboratory indicates that fructose does not have a similar effect in the hippocampi of rats. Specifically, we found that feeding rats a 60% fructose diet for 19 weeks did not affect total IR-β subunit or total Akt/PKB protein, nor the degree of insulin-stimulated phosphorylation of these proteins in the hippocampus [90, 91]. Although we did not measure hippocampal insulin concentrations, it is not likely that the fructose diet reduced hippocampal insulin concentrations. This is because previous studies indicate that a high fructose diet does not reduce peripheral insulin concentrations [62, 92, 93] and the majority of brain insulin concentrations is believed to come from the periphery (reviewed in [94]). One possible reason why we may not have replicated the finding that a 60% fructose diet decreases insulin-stimulated phosphorylation of IR-β and Akt/PKB proteins [42] is that we used hippocampal slices rather than whole brain slices. That possibility does not seem likely, however, given that Mielke and colleagues also found that the high fructose diet impairs other measures of insulin function specifically in hippocampal neurons (decreased protein tyrosine phosphatase and decreased insulin-stimulated LTD). The fact that we studied rats rather than hamsters may account for why we did not replicate these findings. Although both are rodents, rats and hamsters do have differences in energy metabolism and regulation. For instance, hamsters absorb fructose more rapidly than rats [95]. Also, intra-hypothalamic injections of cholecystokinin reduce food intake in rats, but not in hamsters [96, 97]. Rats and hamsters differ in a variety of other ways as well, such as in the concentrations of hypothalamic catecholamines [98], the inflammatory response to a pulmonary toxic insult [99, 100], and cholesterol metabolism in cultured hepatic cells [101]. Regardless of the exact reasons for these differences, our findings suggest that hippocampal insulin resistance does not mediate the memory-impairing effects of a high-fructose diet in rats.

A high fructose diet also may impair memory by disrupting liver function. Feeding rats a 60% fructose diet is a model of NAFLD, which includes hepatomegaly [18], hypertriglyceridemia [18, 37], and increased hepatic lipids [37]. NAFLD encompasses conditions ranging from simple hepatic lipid accumulation to severe hepatic cirrhosis [102]. Humans with NAFLD consume significantly more fructose than do humans without NAFLD [63, 103]. Approximately 50% of people with NAFLD also have cognitive impairments, ranging from mild to severe [104]. Furthermore, patients suffering from liver cirrhosis experience enhanced cognitive performance following a liver transplant [105]. Interesting to note, however, is that in our study a high fructose diet produced NAFLD in female rats [90], but did not impair their memory [66]. This may indicate that NAFLD may not be the mechanism through which a high fructose diet impairs memory, or that females have a mechanism (e.g., estrogen) that protects them from the memory-impairing effects of NAFLD.

Another possibility is that fructose impairs memory by interfering with hippocampal neurogenesis. The dentate gyrus region of the hippocampus is one of only two brain areas in which new neurons are created throughout the lifespan [106-108]. Interestingly, high fructose diets decrease cell proliferation in the hippocampus [47]. In addition, when hippocampal neurogenesis is pharmacologically prevented [109], spatial learning is not affected, but memory is impaired in the water maze task, which suggests that new neurons are essential for the storage and/or retrieval of spatial memories. This pattern of effects (i.e., spared acquisition; impaired retention) parallels the effects of fructose in our studies [18].

Finally, fructose could impair brain function through a process that involves neuroinflammation. It is well documented that neuroinflammation impairs cognition [110-114]. Also, high fat diets may impair memory, at least in part, via neuroinflammation [115, 116]. Elevated fructose consumption activates NFκB and elevates interleukin-1β and tumor necrosis factor-α in the cerebral cortex of rats [44]. Preliminary evidence from our lab suggests that a high fructose diet impairs memory in rats that have the highest levels of hippocampal glial fibrillary acidic protein, a neuroinflammatory marker [90]. In addition to neuroinflammation, oxidative stress is another possible mechanism through which fructose impairs memory. Oxidative stress and inflammatory processes often occur in tandem during cellular dysfunction [117, 118]. Elevated levels of oxidative stress are associated with impaired cognition [119-121], and antioxidant treatment attenuates cognitive impairments [122-124]. High fat diets and high fat/high fructose diets increase hippocampal oxidative stress [79, 125].

PHYSIOLOGICAL RELEVANCE

One question is whether the high fructose concentrations employed in rodent studies are relevant to humans [126, 127], given that the concentrations are much higher than those typically consumed by humans [2, 3]. The differences between rats and humans make it impossible to determine what concentrations are directly comparable between rats and humans based on intake. Although rats are similar to humans, they are not identical in their processing of fructose and lipids [93, 95, 128, 129]. Rats often require much higher doses of substances (e.g. analgesics, antidepressants, anxiolytics) than do humans. For instance, approximately 0.3 mg/kg of fluoxetine alleviates anxiety symptoms in a full-grown human, but it takes approximately 10 mg/kg of fluoxetine to alleviate anxiety symptoms in a rat [130, 131]. We can examine relevance to humans by focusing on endpoints rather than on dietary component concentrations. A significant amount of correlational evidence implicates high fructose consumption in the growing rates of insulin resistance, Type 2 diabetes, and heart disease in humans [6, 40, 132-134], all pathologies that a high fructose diet produces in rats. Moreover, comparisons of other endpoints suggest that fructose concentrations used in rodent studies are not extreme. For instance, in humans, only excessive fructose intake increases body weight [135]; whereas, a 60% fructose concentration does not in rats [18, 136]. Similarly, high fructose concentrations produce diarrhea in humans [137]; in contrast, we observe no such changes in rats. A recent study in rhesus monkeys demonstrates that a high fructose diet produces peripheral pathologies (e.g., insulin resistance, metabolic syndrome) similar to those seen in rodent studies [138]. This provides strong evidence to support the physiological relevance to humans of studies that have employed high fructose concentrations.

Conclusion

A high fructose diet produces a variety of peripheral metabolic disruptions, leading to detrimental effects on the brain (e.g., insulin resistance, inflammation, oxidative stress). A high fructose diet impairs hippocampal-dependent memory in male rats but does not do so in female rats. Although the mechanisms through which elevated fructose ingestion impairs memory are not entirely elucidated, possible intermediates include elevated plasma triglyceride concentrations, NAFLD, decreased neurogenesis, neuroinflammation, and oxidative stress. It is important to consider that humans generally do not eat *just* a high fructose diet. Most imbalanced diets contain an excess of both fat and sugar [4]. A more relevant model of diet-induced pathologies may be a high fat/high sucrose diet [139]. Although it is imperative to understand the combined effects of all dietary components on human pathologies, it also is important that we identify the effects of each dietary component individually. Research on high fructose diets has begun to provide some clarity on the role that fructose alone plays in the development of diet-related brain dysfunctions.

References

[1] Hanover, L.M. and J.S. White, Manufacturing, composition, and applications of fructose. *Am J Clin Nutr,* 1993. 58(5 Suppl):724S-732S.

[2] Vos, M.B., J.E. Kimmons, C. Gillespie, J. Welsh, and H.M. Blanck, Dietary fructose consumption among US children and adults: the Third National Health and Nutrition Examination Survey. *Medscape J. Med.,* 2008. 10(7):160.

[3] Marriott, B.P., N. Cole, and E. Lee, National estimates of dietary fructose intake increased from 1977 to 2004 in the United States. *J. Nutr.,* 2009. 139(6):1228S-1235S.

[4] Wells, H.F. and J.C. Buzby, *Dietary Assessment of Major Trends in U.S. Food Consumption, 1970-2005*, in *Economic Research Bulletin No. 33*, E.R. Service, Editor. 2008, United States Department of Agriculture.

[5] Havel, P.J., Dietary fructose: implications for dysregulation of energy homeostasis and lipid/carbohydrate metabolism. *Nutr. Rev.,* 2005. 63(5):133-57.
[6] Bray, G.A., S.J. Nielsen, and B.M. Popkin, Consumption of high-fructose corn syrup in beverages may play a role in the epidemic of obesity. *Am. J. Clin. Nutr.,* 2004. 79(4):537-43.
[7] Putnam, J.J. and J.E. Allshouse, *Food Consumption, Prices, and Expenditures, 1970-1997.* 1999, U.S.D.A., Economic Research Service.
[8] Topping, D.L. and P.A. Mayes, The concentration of fructose, glucose and lactate in the splanchnic blood vessels of rats absorbing fructose. *Nutr. Metab.,* 1971. 13(6):331-8.
[9] Douard, V. and R.P. Ferraris, Regulation of the fructose transporter GLUT5 in health and disease. *Am. J. Physiol. Endocrinol. Metab.,* 2008. 295(2):E227-37.
[10] Basciano, H., L. Federico, and K. Adeli, Fructose, insulin resistance, and metabolic dyslipidemia. *Nutr. Metab. (Lond),* 2005. 2(1):5.
[11] Mayes, P.A., Intermediary metabolism of fructose. *Am. J. Clin. Nutr.,* 1993. 58(5 Suppl):754S-765S.
[12] Bruckdorfer, K.R., I.H. Khan, and J. Yudkin, Fatty acid synthetase activity in the liver and adipose tissue of rats fed with various carbohydrates. *Biochem. J.,* 1972. 129(2):439-46.
[13] Zavaroni, I., Y.D. Chen, and G.M. Reaven, Studies of the mechanism of fructose-induced hypertriglyceridemia in the rat. *Metabolism,* 1982. 31(11):1077-83.
[14] Vrana, A., P. Fabry, and L. Kazdova, Effect of dietary fructose on fatty acid synthesis in adipose tissue and on triglyceride concentration in blood in the rat. *Nutr. Metab.,* 1973. 15(4):305-13.
[15] Curry, D.L., Effects of mannose and fructose on the synthesis and secretion of insulin. *Pancreas,* 1989. 4(1):2-9.
[16] Grant, A.M., M.R. Christie, and S.J. Ashcroft, Insulin release from human pancreatic islets in vitro. *Diabetologia,* 1980. 19(2):114-7.
[17] Michaelis, O.E.t. and B. Szepesi, Effect of various sugars on hepatic glucose-6-phosphate dehydrogenase, malic enzyme and total liver lipid of the rat. *J. Nutr.,* 1973. 103(5):697-705.
[18] Ross, A.P., T.J. Bartness, J.G. Mielke, and M.B. Parent, A high fructose diet impairs spatial memory in male rats. *Neurobiol. Learn Mem.,* 2009. 92(3):410-6.
[19] Kawasaki, T., K. Igarashi, T. Koeda, K. Sugimoto, K. Nakagawa, S. Hayashi, R. Yamaji, H. Inui, T. Fukusato, and T. Yamanouchi, Rats fed fructose-enriched diets have characteristics of nonalcoholic hepatic steatosis. *J. Nutr.,* 2009. 139(11):2067-71.
[20] Stanhope, K.L., A.A. Bremer, V. Medici, K. Nakajima, Y. Ito, T. Nakano, G. Chen, T.H. Fong, V. Lee, R.I. Menorca, N.L. Keim, and P.J. Havel, Consumption of fructose and high fructose corn syrup increase postprandial triglycerides, LDL-cholesterol, and apolipoprotein-B in young men and women. *J. Clin. Endocrinol. Metab.,* 2011. 96(10):E1596-605.
[21] Bergheim, I., S. Weber, M. Vos, S. Kramer, V. Volynets, S. Kaserouni, C.J. McClain, and S.C. Bischoff, Antibiotics protect against fructose-induced hepatic lipid accumulation in mice: role of endotoxin. *J. Hepatol.,* 2008. 48(6):983-92.

[22] Alzamendi, A., D. Castrogiovanni, H.H. Ortega, R.C. Gaillard, A. Giovambattista, and E. Spinedi, Parametrial adipose tissue and metabolic dysfunctions induced by fructose-rich diet in normal and neonatal-androgenized adult female rats. *Obesity (Silver Spring),* 2010. 18(3):441-8.

[23] Alzamendi, A., A. Giovambattista, A. Raschia, V. Madrid, R.C. Gaillard, O. Rebolledo, J.J. Gagliardino, and E. Spinedi, Fructose-rich diet-induced abdominal adipose tissue endocrine dysfunction in normal male rats. *Endocrine,* 2009. 35(2):227-32.

[24] Zakula, Z., G. Koricanac, S. Tepavcevic, M. Stojiljkovic, T. Milosavljevic, and E.R. Isenovic, Impairment of cardiac insulin signaling in fructose-fed ovariectomized female Wistar rats. *Eur. J. Nutr.,* 2011.

[25] Lee, W.C., C.T. Chien, H.J. Yu, and S.W. Lee, Bladder dysfunction in rats with metabolic syndrome induced by long-term fructose feeding. *J. Urol.,* 2008. 179(6):2470-6.

[26] Kanarek, R.B. and N. Orthen-Gambill, Differential effects of sucrose, fructose and glucose on carbohydrate-induced obesity in rats. *J. Nutr.,* 1982. 112(8):1546-54.

[27] Zavaroni, I., S. Sander, S. Scott, and G.M. Reaven, Effect of fructose feeding on insulin secretion and insulin action in the rat. *Metabolism,* 1980. 29(10):970-3.

[28] Hill, R., N. Baker, and I.L. Chaikoff, Altered metabolic patterns induced in the normal rat by feeding an adequate diet containing fructose as sole carbohydrate. *J. Biol. Chem.,* 1954. 209(2):705-16.

[29] Beck-Nielsen, H., O. Pedersen, and H.O. Lindskov, Impaired cellular insulin binding and insulin sensitivity induced by high-fructose feeding in normal subjects. *Am. J. Clin. Nutr.,* 1980. 33(2):273-8.

[30] Hwang, I.S., H. Ho, B.B. Hoffman, and G.M. Reaven, Fructose-induced insulin resistance and hypertension in rats. *Hypertension,* 1987. 10(5):512-6.

[31] Thorburn, A.W., L.H. Storlien, A.B. Jenkins, S. Khouri, and E.W. Kraegen, Fructose-induced in vivo insulin resistance and elevated plasma triglyceride levels in rats. *Am. J. Clin. Nutr.,* 1989. 49(6):1155-63.

[32] D'Angelo, G., A.A. Elmarakby, D.M. Pollock, and D.W. Stepp, Fructose feeding increases insulin resistance but not blood pressure in Sprague-Dawley rats. *Hypertension,* 2005. 46(4):806-11.

[33] Perez-Pozo, S.E., J. Schold, T. Nakagawa, L.G. Sanchez-Lozada, R.J. Johnson, and J.L. Lillo, Excessive fructose intake induces the features of metabolic syndrome in healthy adult men: role of uric acid in the hypertensive response. *Int. J. Obes. (Lond),* 2010. 34(3):454-61.

[34] Cohen, A.M., A. Teitelbaum, and E. Rosenman, Diabetes induced by a high fructose diet. *Metabolism,* 1977. 26(1):17-24.

[35] Patel, J., A. Iyer, and L. Brown, Evaluation of the chronic complications of diabetes in a high fructose diet in rats. *Indian J. Biochem. Biophys.,* 2009. 46(1):66-72.

[36] Castro, G.S., J.F. Cardoso, H. Vannucchi, S. Zucoloto, and A.A. Jordao, Fructose and NAFLD: metabolic implications and models of induction in rats. *Acta Cir. Bras.,* 2011. 26 Suppl 2:45-50.

[37] Ackerman, Z., M. Oron-Herman, M. Grozovski, T. Rosenthal, O. Pappo, G. Link, and B.A. Sela, Fructose-induced fatty liver disease: hepatic effects of blood pressure and plasma triglyceride reduction. *Hypertension,* 2005. 45(5):1012-8.

[38] Catena, C., G. Giacchetti, M. Novello, G. Colussi, A. Cavarape, and L.A. Sechi, Cellular mechanisms of insulin resistance in rats with fructose-induced hypertension. *Am. J. Hypertens,* 2003. 16(11 Pt 1):973-8.

[39] Hininger-Favier, I., R. Benaraba, S. Coves, R.A. Anderson, and A.M. Roussel, Green tea extract decreases oxidative stress and improves insulin sensitivity in an animal model of insulin resistance, the fructose-fed rat. *J. Am. Coll. Nutr.,* 2009. 28(4):355-61.

[40] Elliott, S.S., N.L. Keim, J.S. Stern, K. Teff, and P.J. Havel, Fructose, weight gain, and the insulin resistance syndrome. *Am. J. Clin. Nutr.,* 2002. 76(5):911-22.

[41] Nandhini, A.T., V. Thirunavukkarasu, M.K. Ravichandran, and C.V. Anuradha, Effect of taurine on biomarkers of oxidative stress in tissues of fructose-fed insulin-resistant rats. *Singapore Med. J.,* 2005. 46(2):82-7.

[42] Mielke, J.G., C. Taghibiglou, L. Liu, Y. Zhang, Z. Jia, K. Adeli, and Y.T. Wang, A biochemical and functional characterization of diet-induced brain insulin resistance. *J. Neurochem.,* 2005. 93(6):1568-78.

[43] Shapiro, A., W. Mu, C. Roncal, K.Y. Cheng, R.J. Johnson, and P.J. Scarpace, Fructose-induced leptin resistance exacerbates weight gain in response to subsequent high-fat feeding. *Am. J. Physiol. Regul. Integr. Comp. Physiol.,* 2008. 295(5):R1370-5.

[44] Liu, X., D. Luo, M. Zheng, Y. Hao, L. Hou, and S. Zhang, Effect of pioglitazone on insulin resistance in fructose-drinking rats correlates with AGEs/RAGE inhibition and block of NADPH oxidase and NF kappa B activation. *Eur. J. Pharmacol.,* 2010. 629(1-3):153-8.

[45] O'Neill, L.A. and C. Kaltschmidt, NF-kappa B: a crucial transcription factor for glial and neuronal cell function. *Trends Neurosci.,* 1997. 20(6):252-8.

[46] Lawrence, T., The nuclear factor NF-kappaB pathway in inflammation. *Cold Spring Harb. Perspect. Biol.,* 2009. 1(6):a001651.

[47] van der Borght, K., R. Kohnke, N. Goransson, T. Deierborg, P. Brundin, C. Erlanson-Albertsson, and A. Lindqvist, Reduced neurogenesis in the rat hippocampus following high fructose consumption. *Regul. Pept.,* 2011. 167(1):26-30.

[48] Luo, D., X. Hou, L. Hou, M. Wang, S. Xu, C. Dong, and X. Liu, Effect of pioglitazone on altered expression of Abeta metabolism-associated molecules in the brain of fructose-drinking rats, a rodent model of insulin resistance. *Eur. J. Pharmacol.,* 2011. 664(1-3):14-9.

[49] Ergorul, C. and H. Eichenbaum, The hippocampus and memory for "what," "where," and "when". *Learn Mem.,* 2004. 11(4):397-405.

[50] Park, C.R., Cognitive effects of insulin in the central nervous system. *Neurosci. Biobehav. Rev.,* 2001. 25(4):311-23.

[51] Convit, A., Links between cognitive impairment in insulin resistance: an explanatory model. *Neurobiol. Aging,* 2005. 26 Suppl 1:31-5.

[52] Messier, C., Impact of impaired glucose tolerance and type 2 diabetes on cognitive aging. *Neurobiol. Aging,* 2005. 26 Suppl 1:26-30.

[53] Stewart, R. and D. Liolitsa, Type 2 diabetes mellitus, cognitive impairment and dementia. *Diabet Med.,* 1999. 16(2):93-112.

[54] Strachan, M.W., I.J. Deary, F.M. Ewing, and B.M. Frier, Is type II diabetes associated with an increased risk of cognitive dysfunction? A critical review of published studies. *Diabetes Care,* 1997. 20(3):438-45.

[55] Zhao, W., H. Chen, H. Xu, E. Moore, N. Meiri, M.J. Quon, and D.L. Alkon, Brain insulin receptors and spatial memory. Correlated changes in gene expression, tyrosine phosphorylation, and signaling molecules in the hippocampus of water maze trained rats. *J. Biol. Chem.,* 1999. 274(49):34893-902.
[56] Dou, J.T., M. Chen, F. Dufour, D.L. Alkon, and W.Q. Zhao, Insulin receptor signaling in long-term memory consolidation following spatial learning. *Learn Mem.,* 2005. 12(6):646-55.
[57] McNay, E.C., C.T. Ong, R.J. McCrimmon, J. Cresswell, J.S. Bogan, and R.S. Sherwin, Hippocampal memory processes are modulated by insulin and high-fat-induced insulin resistance. *Neurobiology of Learning and Memory,* 2010. In Press, Uncorrected Proof.
[58] Moosavi, M., N. Naghdi, N. Maghsoudi, and S. Zahedi Asl, The effect of intrahippocampal insulin microinjection on spatial learning and memory. *Horm. Behav.,* 2006. 50(5):748-52.
[59] Babri, S., H. Gholamipour, S.N. Rad, and S. Khameneh. *Evaluation of insulin intrahippocampal injection on memory consolidation in normal and diabetic male rats.* in *Long-Term Potentiation: Forty Unforgettable Years.* 2006. Atlanta, GA.
[60] Moser, E., M.B. Moser, and P. Andersen, Spatial learning impairment parallels the magnitude of dorsal hippocampal lesions, but is hardly present following ventral lesions. *J. Neurosci.,* 1993. 13(9):3916-25.
[61] Morris, R.G., F. Schenk, F. Tweedie, and L.E. Jarrard, Ibotenate Lesions of Hippocampus and/or Subiculum: Dissociating Components of Allocentric Spatial Learning. *Eur. J. Neurosci.,* 1990. 2(12):1016-1028.
[62] Ross, A.P., E.C. Bruggeman, A.Kasumu, J.G. Mielke, and M.B. Parent, Non-alcoholic fatty liver disease impairs hippocampal-dependent memory in male rats. *Physiol Behav,* 2012. In Press.
[63] Jordan, J.E., S.A. Simandle, C.D. Tulbert, D.W. Busija, and A.W. Miller, Fructose-fed rats are protected against ischemia/reperfusion injury. *J. Pharmacol. Exp. Ther.,* 2003. 307(3):1007-11.
[64] Joyeux-Faure, M., E. Rossini, C. Ribuot, and P. Faure, Fructose-fed rat hearts are protected against ischemia-reperfusion injury. *Exp. Biol. Med. (Maywood),* 2006. 231(4):456-62.
[65] Messier, C., K. Whately, J. Liang, L. Du, and D. Puissant, The effects of a high-fat, high-fructose, and combination diet on learning, weight, and glucose regulation in C57BL/6 mice. *Behav. Brain Res.,* 2007. 178(1):139-45.
[66] Bruggeman, E.C., C. Li, A.P. Ross, J.M. Doherty, B.F. Williams, K.J. Frantz, and M.B. Parent, A high fructose diet does not affect amphetamine self-administration or spatial water maze learning and memory in female rats. *Pharmacol. Biochem. Behav.,* 2011. 99(3):356-64.
[67] Klein, J.R., R. Hurwitz, and N.S. Olsen, Distribution of intravenously injected fructose and glucose between blood and brain. *J. Biol. Chem.,* 1946. 164(2):509-12.
[68] Thurston, J.H., C.A. Levy, S.K. Warren, and E.M. Jones, Permeability of the blood-brain barrier to fructose and the anaerobic use of fructose in the brains of young mice. *J. Neurochem.,* 1972. 19(7):1685-96.
[69] Oldendorf, W.H., Brain uptake of radiolabeled amino acids, amines, and hexoses after arterial injection. *Am. J. Physiol.,* 1971. 221(6):1629-39.

[70] Funari, V.A., J.E. Crandall, and D.R. Tolan, Fructose metabolism in the cerebellum. *Cerebellum,* 2007. 6(2):130-40.

[71] Payne, J., F. Maher, I. Simpson, L. Mattice, and P. Davies, Glucose transporter Glut 5 expression in microglial cells. *Glia,* 1997. 21(3):327-31.

[72] Shu, H.J., K. Isenberg, R.J. Cormier, A. Benz, and C.F. Zorumski, Expression of fructose sensitive glucose transporter in the brains of fructose-fed rats. *Neuroscience,* 2006. 140(3):889-95.

[73] Purnell, J.Q., B.A. Klopfenstein, A.A. Stevens, P.J. Havel, S.H. Adams, T.N. Dunn, C. Krisky, and W.D. Rooney, Brain functional magnetic resonance imaging response to glucose and fructose infusions in humans. *Diabetes Obes. Metab.,* 2011. 13(3):229-34.

[74] Winocur, G. and C.E. Greenwood, The effects of high fat diets and environmental influences on cognitive performance in rats. *Behav. Brain Res.,* 1999. 101(2):153-61.

[75] Farr, S.A., K.A. Yamada, D.A. Butterfield, H.M. Abdul, L. Xu, N.E. Miller, W.A. Banks, and J.E. Morley, Obesity and hypertriglyceridemia produce cognitive impairment. *Endocrinology,* 2008. 149(5):2628-36.

[76] Granholm, A.C., H.A. Bimonte-Nelson, A.B. Moore, M.E. Nelson, L.R. Freeman, and K. Sambamurti, Effects of a saturated fat and high cholesterol diet on memory and hippocampal morphology in the middle-aged rat. *J. Alzheimers Dis.,* 2008. 14(2):133-45.

[77] Couchepin, C., K.A. Le, M. Bortolotti, J.A. da Encarnacao, J.B. Oboni, C. Tran, P. Schneiter, and L. Tappy, Markedly blunted metabolic effects of fructose in healthy young female subjects compared with male subjects. *Diabetes Care,* 2008. 31(6):1254-6.

[78] Galipeau, D., S. Verma, and J.H. McNeill, Female rats are protected against fructose-induced changes in metabolism and blood pressure. *Am. J. Physiol. Heart Circ. Physiol.,* 2002. 283(6):H2478-84.

[79] Stranahan, A.M., R.G. Cutler, C. Button, R. Telljohann, and M.P. Mattson, Diet-induced elevations in serum cholesterol are associated with alterations in hippocampal lipid metabolism and increased oxidative stress. *J. Neurochem.,* 2011. 118(4):611-5.

[80] Malaisse, W.J., Y. Zhang, K. Louchami, A. Sener, L. Portois, and Y.A. Carpentier, Brain phospholipid and triglyceride fatty acid content and pattern in Type 1 and Type 2 diabetic rats. *Neurosci. Lett.,* 2006. 409(1):75-9.

[81] Cotera, V.E., E. Jorge, and E.C. Mcnay, *Saturated fatty acids impair, while unsaturated fatty acids enhance, hippocampal memory and metabolic processes*. 2010, Society for Neuroscience: San Diego.

[82] Lynch, M.A., Long-term potentiation and memory. *Physiol. Rev.,* 2004. 84(1):87-136.

[83] Banks, W.A., A.B. Coon, S.M. Robinson, A. Moinuddin, J.M. Shultz, R. Nakaoke, and J.E. Morley, Triglycerides induce leptin resistance at the blood-brain barrier. *Diabetes,* 2004. 53(5):1253-60.

[84] Paz-Filho, G.J., T. Babikian, R. Asarnow, T. Delibasi, K. Esposito, H.K. Erol, M.L. Wong, and J. Licinio, Leptin replacement improves cognitive development. *PLoS One,* 2008. 3(8):e3098.

[85] Farr, S.A., W.A. Banks, and J.E. Morley, Effects of leptin on memory processing. *Peptides,* 2006. 27(6):1420-5.

[86] Oomura, Y., N. Hori, T. Shiraishi, K. Fukunaga, H. Takeda, M. Tsuji, T. Matsumiya, M. Ishibashi, S. Aou, X.L. Li, D. Kohno, K. Uramura, H. Sougawa, T. Yada, M.J. Wayner, and K. Sasaki, Leptin facilitates learning and memory performance and enhances hippocampal CA1 long-term potentiation and CaMK II phosphorylation in rats. *Peptides,* 2006. 27(11):2738-49.

[87] Dietrich, M.O., A. Muller, M. Bolos, E. Carro, M.L. Perry, L.V. Portela, D.O. Souza, and I. Torres-Aleman, Western style diet impairs entrance of blood-borne insulin-like growth factor-1 into the brain. *Neuromolecular Med.,* 2007. 9(4):324-30.

[88] Lupien, S.B., E.J. Bluhm, and D.N. Ishii, Systemic insulin-like growth factor-I administration prevents cognitive impairment in diabetic rats, and brain IGF regulates learning/memory in normal adult rats. *J. Neurosci. Res.,* 2003. 74(4):512-23.

[89] Aleman, A., W.R. de Vries, E.H. de Haan, H.J. Verhaar, M.M. Samson, and H.P. Koppeschaar, Age-sensitive cognitive function, growth hormone and insulin-like growth factor 1 plasma levels in healthy older men. *Neuropsychobiology,* 2000. 41(2):73-8.

[90] Bruggeman, E.C. Unpublished.

[91] Ross, A.P. Unpublished.

[92] Zaman, M.Q., V. Leray, J. Le Bloc'h, C. Thorin, K. Ouguerram, and P. Nguyen, Lipid profile and insulin sensitivity in rats fed with high-fat or high-fructose diets. *Br. J. Nutr.,* 2011. 106 Suppl 1:S206-10.

[93] Taghibiglou, C., A. Carpentier, S.C. Van Iderstine, B. Chen, D. Rudy, A. Aiton, G.F. Lewis, and K. Adeli, Mechanisms of hepatic very low density lipoprotein overproduction in insulin resistance. Evidence for enhanced lipoprotein assembly, reduced intracellular ApoB degradation, and increased microsomal triglyceride transfer protein in a fructose-fed hamster model. *J. Biol. Chem.,* 2000. 275(12):8416-25.

[94] Mielke, J.G. and Y.T. Wang, Insulin, synaptic function, and opportunities for neuroprotection. *Prog. Mol. Biol. Transl. Sci.,* 2011. 98:133-86.

[95] Thomson, A.B., C.A. Hotke, and W.M. Weinstein, Comparison of kinetic constants of hexose uptake in four animal species and man. *Comp. Biochem. Physiol. A Comp. Physiol.,* 1982. 72(1):225-36.

[96] Miceli, M.O. and C.W. Malsbury, Feeding and drinking responses in the golden hamster following treatment with cholecystokinin and angiotensin II. *Peptides,* 1983. 4(1):103-6.

[97] Chen, J., K.A. Scott, Z. Zhao, T.H. Moran, and S. Bi, Characterization of the feeding inhibition and neural activation produced by dorsomedial hypothalamic cholecystokinin administration. *Neuroscience,* 2008. 152(1):178-88.

[98] Fuller, R.W. and S.K. Hemrick-Luecke, Species differences in epinephrine concentration and norepinephrine N-methyltransferase activity in hypothalamus and brain stem. *Comp. Biochem. Physiol. C,* 1983. 74(1):47-9.

[99] Carter, J.M. and K.E. Driscoll, The role of inflammation, oxidative stress, and proliferation in silica-induced lung disease: a species comparison. *J. Environ. Pathol. Toxicol. Oncol.,* 2001. 20 Suppl 1:33-43.

[100] Dorger, M., A.M. Allmeling, R. Kiefmann, S. Munzing, K. Messmer, and F. Krombach, Early inflammatory response to asbestos exposure in rat and hamster lungs: role of inducible nitric oxide synthase. *Toxicol. Appl. Pharmacol.,* 2002. 181(2):93-105.

[101] Botham, K.M., V.Q. Hoang, A.K. Jones, M.J. Martinez, B. Ochoa, and K.E. Suckling, Comparison of the effects of cyclic AMP analogues on cholesterol metabolism in cultured rat and hamster hepatocytes. *Comp. Biochem. Physiol. B Biochem. Mol. Biol.,* 1996. 113(1):185-91.

[102] Kopec, K.L. and D. Burns, Nonalcoholic fatty liver disease: a review of the spectrum of disease, diagnosis, and therapy. *Nutr. Clin. Pract.,* 2011. 26(5):565-76.

[103] Thuy, S., R. Ladurner, V. Volynets, S. Wagner, S. Strahl, A. Konigsrainer, K.P. Maier, S.C. Bischoff, and I. Bergheim, Nonalcoholic fatty liver disease in humans is associated with increased plasma endotoxin and plasminogen activator inhibitor 1 concentrations and with fructose intake. *J. Nutr.,* 2008. 138(8):1452-5.

[104] Newton, J.L., Systemic symptoms in non-alcoholic fatty liver disease. *Dig. Dis.,* 2010. 28(1):214-9.

[105] Garcia-Martinez, R. and J. Cordoba, Acute-on-chronic liver failure: the brain. *Curr. Opin. Crit. Care,* 2011. 17(2):177-83.

[106] Eriksson, P.S., E. Perfilieva, T. Bjork-Eriksson, A.M. Alborn, C. Nordborg, D.A. Peterson, and F.H. Gage, Neurogenesis in the adult human hippocampus. *Nat. Med.,* 1998. 4(11):1313-7.

[107] Lledo, P.M., M. Alonso, and M.S. Grubb, Adult neurogenesis and functional plasticity in neuronal circuits. *Nat. Rev. Neurosci.,* 2006. 7(3):179-93.

[108] Gould, E., A. Beylin, P. Tanapat, A. Reeves, and T.J. Shors, Learning enhances adult neurogenesis in the hippocampal formation. *Nat. Neurosci.,* 1999. 2(3):260-5.

[109] Shors, T.J., D.A. Townsend, M. Zhao, Y. Kozorovitskiy, and E. Gould, Neurogenesis may relate to some but not all types of hippocampal-dependent learning. *Hippocampus,* 2002. 12(5):578-84.

[110] Oitzl, M.S., H. van Oers, B. Schobitz, and E.R. de Kloet, Interleukin-1 beta, but not interleukin-6, impairs spatial navigation learning. *Brain Res.,* 1993. 613(1):160-3.

[111] Lee, J.W., Y.K. Lee, D.Y. Yuk, D.Y. Choi, S.B. Ban, K.W. Oh, and J.T. Hong, Neuro-inflammation induced by lipopolysaccharide causes cognitive impairment through enhancement of beta-amyloid generation. *J. Neuroinflammation,* 2008. 5:37.

[112] Tanaka, S., M. Ide, T. Shibutani, H. Ohtaki, S. Numazawa, S. Shioda, and T. Yoshida, Lipopolysaccharide-induced microglial activation induces learning and memory deficits without neuronal cell death in rats. *J. Neurosci. Res.,* 2006. 83(4):557-66.

[113] Hauss-Wegrzyniak, B., M.G. Vannucchi, and G.L. Wenk, Behavioral and ultrastructural changes induced by chronic neuroinflammation in young rats. *Brain Res.,* 2000. 859(1):157-66.

[114] Hauss-Wegrzyniak, B., P. Dobrzanski, J.D. Stoehr, and G.L. Wenk, Chronic neuro-inflammation in rats reproduces components of the neurobiology of Alzheimer's disease. *Brain Res.,* 1998. 780(2):294-303.

[115] Lu, J., D.M. Wu, Y.L. Zheng, B. Hu, W. Cheng, Z.F. Zhang, and Q. Shan, Ursolic acid improves high fat diet-induced cognitive impairments by blocking endoplasmic reticulum stress and IkappaB kinase beta/nuclear factor-kappaB-mediated inflammatory pathways in mice. *Brain Behav. Immun,* 2011. 25(8):1658-67.

[116] Pistell, P.J., C.D. Morrison, S. Gupta, A.G. Knight, J.N. Keller, D.K. Ingram, and A.J. Bruce-Keller, Cognitive impairment following high fat diet consumption is associated with brain inflammation. *Journal of Neuroimmunology,* 2010. 219(1-2):25-32.

[117] Zhang, K., Integration of ER stress, oxidative stress and the inflammatory response in health and disease. *Int. J. Clin. Exp. Med.,* 2010. 3(1):33-40.

[118] Flohe, L., R. Brigelius-Flohe, C. Saliou, M.G. Traber, and L. Packer, Redox regulation of NF-kappa B activation. *Free Radic. Biol. Med.,* 1997. 22(6):1115-26.

[119] Massaad, C.A. and E. Klann, Reactive oxygen species in the regulation of synaptic plasticity and memory. *Antioxid. Redox. Signal,* 2011. 14(10):2013-54.

[120] Sultana, R., M. Perluigi, and D.A. Butterfield, Oxidatively modified proteins in Alzheimer's disease (AD), mild cognitive impairment and animal models of AD: role of Abeta in pathogenesis. *Acta Neuropathol.,* 2009. 118(1):131-50.

[121] Lovell, M.A. and W.R. Markesbery, Oxidative DNA damage in mild cognitive impairment and late-stage Alzheimer's disease. *Nucleic Acids Res.,* 2007. 35(22):7497-504.

[122] Head, E., Oxidative damage and cognitive dysfunction: antioxidant treatments to promote healthy brain aging. *Neurochem. Res.,* 2009. 34(4):670-8.

[123] Mecocci, P., Oxidative stress in mild cognitive impairment and Alzheimer disease: a continuum. *J. Alzheimers Dis.,* 2004. 6(2):159-63.

[124] Alzoubi, K.H., O.F. Khabour, B.A. Rashid, I.M. Damaj, and H.A. Salah, The neuroprotective effect of vitamin E on chronic sleep deprivation-induced memory impairment: the role of oxidative stress. *Behav. Brain Res.,* 2012. 226(1):205-10.

[125] Morrison, C.D., P.J. Pistell, D.K. Ingram, W.D. Johnson, Y. Liu, S.O. Fernandez-Kim, C.L. White, M.N. Purpera, R.M. Uranga, A.J. Bruce-Keller, and J.N. Keller, High fat diet increases hippocampal oxidative stress and cognitive impairment in aged mice: implications for decreased Nrf2 signaling. *J. Neurochem.,* 2010. 114(6):1581-9.

[126] Dolan, L.C., S.M. Potter, and G.A. Burdock, Evidence-based review on the effect of normal dietary consumption of fructose on blood lipids and body weight of overweight and obese individuals. *Crit. Rev. Food Sci. Nutr.,* 2010. 50(10):889-918.

[127] Rizkalla, S.W., Health implications of fructose consumption: A review of recent data. *Nutr. Metab. (Lond),* 2010. 7:82.

[128] Adams, S.H., K.L. Stanhope, R.W. Grant, B.P. Cummings, and P.J. Havel, Metabolic and endocrine profiles in response to systemic infusion of fructose and glucose in rhesus macaques. *Endocrinology,* 2008. 149(6):3002-8.

[129] Masson, S., O. Henriksen, A. Stengaard, C. Thomsen, and B. Quistorff, Hepatic metabolism during constant infusion of fructose; comparative studies with 31P-magnetic resonance spectroscopy in man and rats. *Biochim. Biophys. Acta,* 1994. 1199(2):166-74.

[130] Eli-Lilly. *PROZAC Prescribing Information.* 1987 revised March 19, 2009 June 17, 2009]; Available from: http://pi.lilly.com/us/prozac. pdf?reqNacId=undefined.

[131] Borsini, F., J. Podhorna, and D. Marazziti, Do animal models of anxiety predict anxiolytic-like effects of antidepressants? *Psychopharmacology (Berl),* 2002. 163(2):121-41.

[132] Gross, L.S., L. Li, E.S. Ford, and S. Liu, Increased consumption of refined carbohydrates and the epidemic of type 2 diabetes in the United States: an ecologic assessment. *Am. J. Clin. Nutr.,* 2004. 79(5):774-9.

[133] Hu, F.B. and V.S. Malik, Sugar-sweetened beverages and risk of obesity and type 2 diabetes: epidemiologic evidence. *Physiol. Behav.,* 2010. 100(1):47-54.

[134] Montonen, J., R. Jarvinen, P. Knekt, M. Heliovaara, and A. Reunanen, Consumption of sweetened beverages and intakes of fructose and glucose predict type 2 diabetes occurrence. *Journal of Nutrition,* 2007. 137(6):1447-1454.

[135] Livesey, G. and R. Taylor, Fructose consumption and consequences for glycation, plasma triacylglycerol, and body weight: meta-analyses and meta-regression models of intervention studies. *Am. J. Clin. Nutr.,* 2008. 88(5):1419-37.

[136] Abdullah, M.M., N.N. Riediger, Q. Chen, Z. Zhao, N. Azordegan, Z. Xu, G. Fischer, R.A. Othman, G.N. Pierce, P.S. Tappia, J. Zou, and M.H. Moghadasian, Effects of long-term consumption of a high-fructose diet on conventional cardiovascular risk factors in Sprague-Dawley rats. *Mol. Cell Biochem.,* 2009. 327(1-2):247-56.

[137] Skoog, S.M. and A.E. Bharucha, Dietary fructose and gastrointestinal symptoms: a review. *Am. J. Gastroenterol.,* 2004. 99(10):2046-50.

[138] Bremer, A.A., K.L. Stanhope, J.L. Graham, B.P. Cummings, W. Wang, B.R. Saville, and P.J. Havel, Fructose-fed rhesus monkeys: a nonhuman primate model of insulin resistance, metabolic syndrome, and type 2 diabetes. *Clin. Transl. Sci.,* 2011. 4(4):243-52.

[139] Sampey, B.P., A.M. Vanhoose, H.M. Winfield, A.J. Freemerman, M.J. Muehlbauer, P.T. Fueger, C.B. Newgard, and L. Makowski, Cafeteria diet is a robust model of human metabolic syndrome with liver and adipose inflammation: comparison to high-fat diet. *Obesity (Silver Spring),* 2011. 19(6):1109-17.

In: Fructose
Editors: Brandon M. Johnston and Aaron B. Collins
ISBN: 978-1-62081-126-9

Chapter 5

ROLE OF FRUCTOSE IN BODY FUNCTIONS: AN OVERVIEW

N. Assy,[1*] F. Adawi[2], and W. Nseir[3]
[1]Liver Unit, Ziv Medical Center, Safed, Israel.
Bar-Ilan University, Safed, Israel
[2]Endocrinology Unit, Ziv Medical Center, Safed, Israel
[3]Department of Internal Medicine, Holy Family Hospital,
Nazareth, Israel

ABSTRACT

The consumption of fructose has increased considerably in the world during the last decades. Excessive fructose consumption may be responsible in part for the increasing prevalence of obesity, non alcoholic fatty liver disease (NAFLD), metabolic syndrome, and diabetes mellitus. Fructose promotes the formation of toxic advanced glycation end-products (AGE'S), which appear to play a role in the development of atherosclerosis, aging process; and in the pathogenesis of vascular, renal and ocular complication of diabetes; Fructose has also been implicated as the main cause of symptoms in some patients with chronic diarrhea or other functional bowel disturbances (IBS). Although the long term effects of fructose consumption have not been adequately studied in humans, the available evidence suggests it may be more harmful than is generally recognized.

INTRODUCTION

High-fructose corn syrup (HFCS) is now used extensively in carbonated beverages and other sweetened drinks, baked goods, candies, canned fruits, jams, jellies, and dairy products. Fructose consumption increased by 50 percent, from 60g/day in 1970 to 120 g/day in 2010[1]. In contrast, intake of naturally occurring fructose from fruits and vegetables is only about 15 g/day. HFCS contains fructose (57% of total calories) and glucose (43% of total

* Corresponding author: Assy Nimer, MD, Liver Unit, Ziv Medical Center, POB 1008, Bar-Ilan University, Safed 13100, Israel, assy.n@ziv.health.gov.il, Phone +97246828441/5. Fax 97246828442.

calories) in their monosaccharide forms. While fructose consumption has not adversely affected glycemic control in most studies [2], fructose has deleterious effects on other aspects of metabolism (Table 1). As a reducing sugar, fructose reacts with protein molecules to form toxic advanced glycation end-products (AGEs), which appear to accelerate the aging process and to play a role in the pathogenesis of diabetes complications and cardiovascular disease. Fructose consumption has been shown to cause hypertriglyceridemia and hyperuricemia and, in individuals consuming a hyper caloric diet, to induce insulin resistance and other precursor of the metabolic syndrome. Fructose has also been implicated as the main cause of symptoms in some patients with chronic diarrhea or other functional bowel disturbances. Finally, there is evidence that excessive fructose consumption is responsible in part for the increasing prevalence of obesity, metabolic syndrome, non-alcoholic fatty liver disease, and type 2 diabetes mellitus [3]. Although the long-term effects of fructose consumption have not been adequately studied in humans, the available evidence suggests it may be more harmful than is generally recognized.

Fructose Synthesis

Fructose is a simple sugar with a chemical formula ($C6H12O6$) similar to that of glucose. In the diet, fructose is consumed in various amounts with fruits, honey, beverages sweetened with HFCS and as a constituent of sucrose.

Absorption of fructose from the intestine into the portal blood is aided by glucose transporter-5 at the brush border and baso lateral membranes of the jejunum then uptake by hepatocytes.

Table 1. Potential Adverse Health Effects of Dietary Fructose

Obesity
Aging
Insulin Resistance
Fatty Liver
Diabetes and its complication
Metabolic Syndrome
Hypertriglyceridemia
Hyperuricemia
Chronic Diarrhea
Irritable bowel syndrome
Urticaria

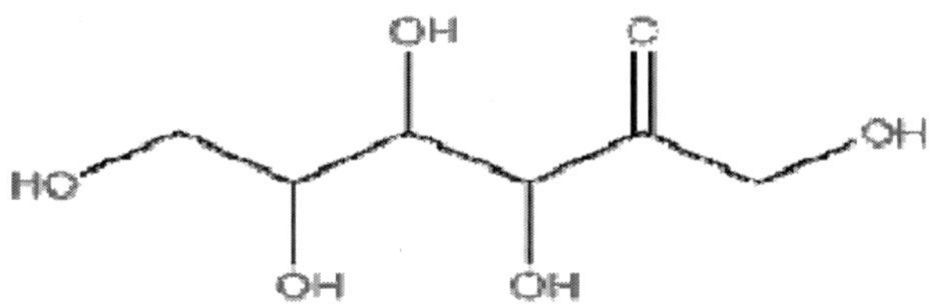

Fructose is phosphorylated by fructokinase, forming fructose-1-phosphate, which can then be converted to several three-carbon molecules, including glyceraldehydes, dihydroxy-acetone phosphate and glyceraldehyde-3-phosphate [Figure 1]. Some of these 3 carbon molecules could be converted to glucose through gluconeogenesis, or they could be used to generate other products such as triglyceride (TG). The second metabolism of fructose, i.e., the extraheptic metabolism that bypasses fructokinase, allows the carbons from fructose to enter glycolysis downstream of this enzyme. The 3 carbon molecules can eventually be used for the synthesis of glycerol and fatty acids, which through esterification can form TGs. The concentration of fructose in fasting blood of healthy humans is typically 1 mg /dl.

After oral administration of fructose load in doses ranging from approximately 18 gr (0.25g/kg of body weight) to 100g, the mean plasma or serum fructose concentration increased in a dose dependant manner, to values ranging from 4.5-13.0 mg/dl and peak fructose concentrations were seen 30-60 minutes after fructose ingestion. A 20-ounce soft drink containing 32.6 g of fructose would therefore be expected to increase the fasting serum fructose concentration by approximately four-fold.

Specific Function of Fructose

Fructose is a simple carbohydrate, or monosaccharide. Fructose is used therapeutically as a nutrient, fluid replenisher, and in table sugar. Fructose has low cost, and high relative sweetness. Simple sugars and carbohydrates are the easiest form of energy for the body, since they are broken down more rapidly than complex foods like proteins, fats and whole grains and vegetables. The body takes these simple sugars and converts them to glucose. Excess glucose is stored as glycogen, and excess glycogen is converted to fat for storage. Fructose can only be metabolized by the liver. Fructose can be converted into glucose by the liver, but this conversion only takes place when large amounts of fructose are consumed after periods of prolonged starvation. Fructose itself cannot be stored as glycogen, although small amounts of fructose do increase the rate at which glucose is converted into glycogen.

Fructose is 7 times more likely than glucose to form advanced glycation end –products (AGE'S). Fructose does not suppress ghrelin and does not stimulate insulin or leptin [4-6].

While moderate amounts of fructose will likely be used to meet the liver's immediate energy needs, large amounts of it are likely to be converted into fat by the liver. Consuming large amounts of fructose could have adverse health effects because fat synthesized by the liver is released as very low density lipoproteins, or VLDL, that greatly increases the risk of coronary artery disease [7]

Health Implication of Fructose

Fructose and Insulin Resistance

Fructose consumption increases postprandial TG concentrations within 24 h [8-9], which suggests that postprandial hypertriglyceridemia is the earliest metabolic perturbation associated with fructose consumption. The most likely mechanism for the postprandial hypertriglyceridemia is increased hepatic de-novo lipogenesis (DNL), which in turn up

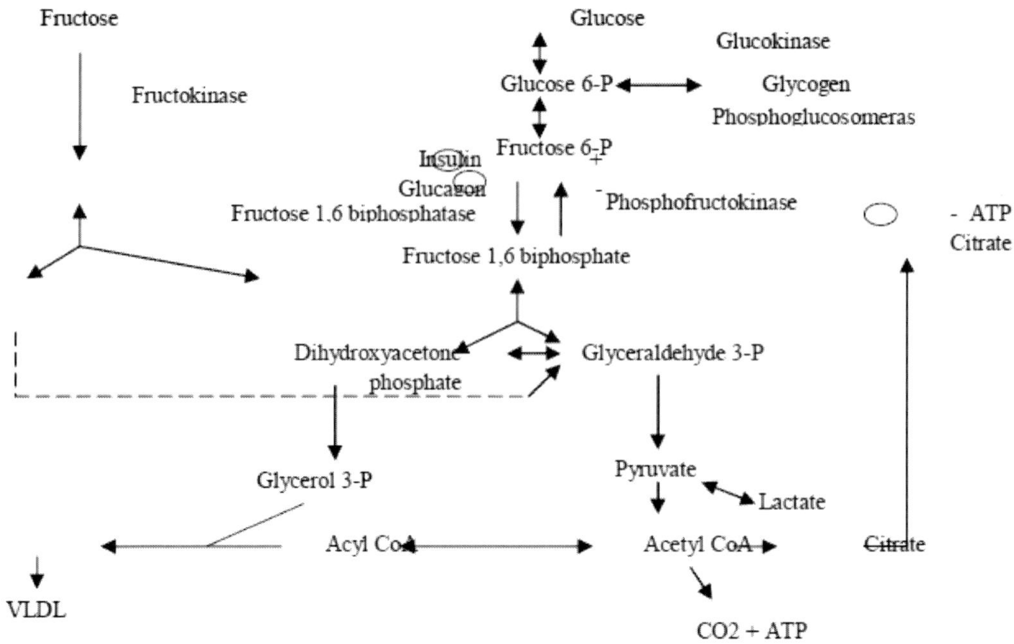

Figure 1.Fructose is phosphorylated by fructokinase, forming fructose-1-phosphate, which can then be converted to several three-carbon molecules, including glyceraldehydes, dihydroxy-acetone phosphate and glyceraldehyde-3-phosphate.

regulates VLDL production and secretion [10]. Fructose consumption can promote hepatic lipogenesis primarily because the liver is the main site of fructose metabolism; secondly, entry of fructose into glycolysis via fructose-1-phosphate bypasses the main rate controlling step of glycolysis catalyzed by phosphor fructokinase, thus providing unregulated amounts of lipogenic substrates acetyl-CoA and glycerol-3-phosphate [10]; thirdly, fructose can activate sterol receptor element binding protein-1c (SREBP-1c) independently of insulin, which then activates fat genes involved in DNL [11,12]. Recently, Stanphone KL demonstrated that consuming fructose-sweetened beverages, not glucose-sweetened beverages increases DNL, promotes dyslipidemia, decreases insulin sensitivity and increases visceral adiposity in overweight and obese adults [13,14]**,** One study of lean women found that 4 days of over feeding with a sucrose-sweetened (glucose + fructose) drink increased de novo lipogenesis by 200-300% [15]. Another feeding study showed that 2 days of high fructose intake (30% of kcal/day, consumed as sweetened beverage at every meal) resulted in decreased postprandial glucose concentration and insulin response and prolonged alimentary lipemia in women [10]. A recent clinical study indicates that NAFLD patients have a higher intake of soft drink and meat and a tendency towards a lower intake of fish rich in omega-3[16].

Fructose and Diabetes Mellitus

Diabetes mellitus type 2 is a direct consequence of lipotoxicity promoting insulin resistance and accelerating pancreatic B-cell failure. Elevated plasma free fatty acids are associated with the progression from pre diabetes (IFG, IGT) to type 2 diabetes mellitus [17]. The presence of diabetes mellitus in patients with NASH have significant clinical implication, as NASH appears to follow a more aggressive course in the presence of hyperglycemia , placing a growing number of diabetic patients at risk of progressive liver disease [17]. In short-term studies in humans, fructose ingestion had no deleterious effect on glucose metabolism. In studies lasting 3-8 days, substitution of sucrose or starch with fructose improved glycemic control in patients with type 1 or type 2 diabetes mellitus. Similarly, no adverse effects of fructose feeding on glycemic control were seen in studies lasting 1-3 months. In a series of patients with diet controlled type 2 diabetes, substitution of sucrose by fructose (13% of calories) for three months had no significant effect on fasting plasma glucose levels or postprandial plasma glucose and insulin responses[17]. Long-term fructose consumption may promote the development of diabetes, even though fructose usually has no adverse effects on glucose tolerance in the short- and intermediate term. In rats, long-term feeding of moderate amounts of fructose (15% of the diet by weight) resulted in impaired glucose tolerance [18] and high-fructose diets (72% by weight) resulted in the development of diabetes mellitus and diffuse glomerulosclerosis [19-20].

Fructose and Obesity

The association between HFCS consumption and obesity is due in part to metabolic changes induced by fructose or HFCS, rather than merely to an increase in total energy intake [21]. In studies in baboons, consumption of sucrose compared with glucose promoted the development of abdominal obesity, suggesting that the fructose moiety of sucrose was responsible for the increase in abdominal fat [22-23]. In addition, some strains of mice showed an increase in visceral fat accumulation when fed a high-fructose diet [24]. Overweight among children has increased dramatically during the past two decades and is approaching epidemic proportions [25, 26]. The results of Dubois et al, study indicated that regular sugar-sweetened beverage consumption, especially between meals, may put children at greater risk for overweight in childhood. Because there is a positive association between consumption of sugar-sweetened beverage and body weight among preschool-aged children, they advise that parents should limit the quantity of such sweetened beverages consumed during preschool years [27]. In the field trial, 644 British schoolchildren (ages 7-11 years) were randomly assigned to a control group or to an education program designed to reduce their consumption of carbonated drinks (both sweetened and unsweetened). The mean consumption of carbonated drinks decreased by 50 ml/day in the intervention group and increased by 16.7 ml/day in the control group. After 12 months, the approximate percentage of overweight and obese children had increased in the control group from 20% to 27.5%, compared with a decrease in the intervention group from 20% to 19.8% [28].

Fructose and Non Alcoholic Fatty Liver (NAFLD)

Risk factors for NAFLD include obesity, type 2 diabetes, insulin resistance and hypertriglyceridemia. Of note, each of these risk factors can occur as a result of excessive fructose consumption. Recently Assy [29-30, Figure 2] et al showed soft drink consumption is linked with fatty liver independently by metabolic syndrome diagnosis. High-fructose diets have induced fatty liver in rats [31] and ducks, [32] such diets have also caused increases in hepatic lipid per oxidation [33] and activation of inflammatory pathways in the liver of rats [34].

Fructose is lipogenic and stimulates TG synthesis [11]. Splanchnic perfusion studies demonstrate that fructose produces higher rates of TG secretion from the liver than equimolar amounts of glucose [35]. The long-term administration of fructose to rats results in hepatic macro- and micro vesicular steatosis with a 198% increase in hepatic TGs and an 89% increase in hepatic cholesterol concentration [36]. Furthermore, the administration of a diet with 25% of total energy as sucrose (which contains 50% fructose) resulted in a rise in hepatic ALT and AST levels within 18 days [37-38].

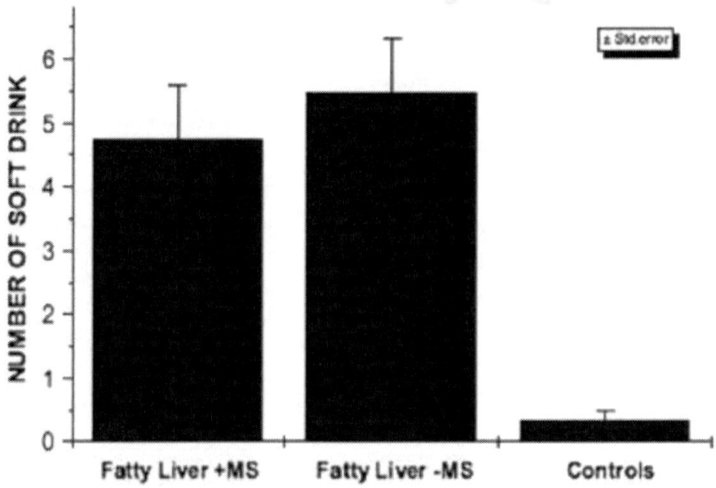

Figure 2. Number of daily soft drinks in non-alcoholic fatty liver disease (NAFLD) patients with or without metabolic syndrome (MS) and in controls. *$P<0.07$; NAFLD without metabolic syndrome versus NAFLD with metabolic syndrome. **$p<0.001$ between NAFLD subgroups and controls.

Indeed, total fructose intake averages approximately 12% of total energy intake and may increase to 15% in some subgroups in the US population [39].Animals maintained on a chronic high fructose diet develop elevated non-esterifed fatty acids (NEFA) and hyper-insulinemia at the expense of glycemic control [19]. This is not surprising, as fructose-induced metabolic dyslipidemia is usually accompanied by whole body insulin resistance [40] and reduced hepatic insulin sensitivity [41]. The metabolism of fructose is distinct from glucose. Before converging with the glycolytic pathway, initial fructose metabolism involves phosphorylation of fructose to fructose-1 phosphate by fructokinase (ketohexokinase, KHK) using the substrate ATP. Unlike glucokinase, the phosphorylation of fructose by fructokinase is specific for fructose and not rate limited. The high activity of fructokinase in phosphorylating fructose to fructose-1- phosphate in the liver, could result in hepatic ATP depletion [39]. Indeed, fructose has been shown to cause ATP depletion in humans [42,43], and recovery from fructose-induced ATP depletion was found to be delayed in subjects with NALFD in studies that used phosphorus-1 magnetic resonance spectroscopy to assess hepatic metabolism [44]. In some respects, fructose-induced ATP depletion resembles hepatic ischemia [45]. In rats, fructose administration increases hepatic lipid peroxidation and activation of inflammatory pathways [33]. Cirrilo et al found that incubation of endothelial cells or renal tubular cells with postprandial concentrations of fructose reduces intracellular ATP and activates proinflammatory and prooxidative responses [46]. Therefore, high fructose consumption may contribute to NAFLD pathogenesis because fructose-induced ATP depletion promotes hepatic necro inflammation. Moreover, fructose promote insulin resistance, lipid peroxidation, dylipidemia, increase arterial blood pressure, increase advanced glycation end products (AGE"S), and increase hepatic inflammation [46]. Ouyang et al found that subjects with NAFLD have a significantly greater intake of sweetened beverages by history, representing 2-fold greater than the mean intake in both controls and in population-based studies. The second finding was that the key initiating enzyme in fructose metabolism, ketohexokinase (fructokinase, KHK), was also increased 2-fold in the liver biopsies of these patients compared to controls [47]. The increase in KHK levels is consistent with the known effect of fructose to up regulate KHK in the liver of rats [48, 49]. Patients on a high fructose or sucrose diet show a greater uric acid response to a bolus of fructose [50, 51] consistent with the up regulation of KHK activity. Finally, uric acid levels can predict the development of NAFLD [52]. There is also increasing evidence that the rise in uric acid may also have a potential role in causing features of the metabolic syndrome [53], in part by the ability of uric acid to deplete endothelial nitric oxide levels [54] and by activating the adipocyte [48].

Fructose and Metabolic Syndrome

Reaven noted that several risk factors (eg, dyslipidemia, hypertension hyperglycemia) commonly cluster together [55]. This clustering he called Syndrome X, and he recognized it as a multiplex risk factor for cardiovascular disease (CVD). Other researchers use the term metabolic syndrome for this clustering of metabolic risk factors. ATP III used this alternative term [56]. Beyond CVD and type 2 diabetes, individuals with metabolic syndrome are susceptible to other conditions, notably polycystic ovary syndrome, fatty liver, cholesterol gallstones, asthma, sleep disturbances, some forms of cancer, and also associated with a pro-inflammatory /prothrombotic state that include elevated levels of C-reactive protein, endothelial dysfunction,hyperfibrogenemia, increased platelet aggregation, increased levels of plasminogen activator, elevated uric acid levels, microalbuminuria, and a shift toward small, dense particles of low–density lipoprotein (LDL) [57] . The major characteristics of metabolic syndrome include insulin resistance, abdominal obesity, elevated blood pressure, and lipid abnormalities (i.e., elevated levels of TGs and low levels of high-density lipoprotein [HDL] cholesterol). The role of fructose in insulin resistance, hyperglycemia, and obesity that constitute important elements of the metabolic syndrome were discussed above [57]. Visceral adipose tissue and dyslipidemia induced by fructose/sucrose consumption play a major role in the development and progression of metabolic syndrome. The main role of adipose tissue is to take up excess fatty acids provided by the diet and to store them in the form of TG to be used as an energy supply for the body in times of starvation, but there is a limited capacity of adipose tissue to store fat. This maximum capacity may be reached in states of obesity, resulting in an impaired ability of adipose tissue to acquire dietary fatty acids and, therefore, increased levels of fatty acids in the circulation [57] Signaling abnormalities in adipocytes can also trigger lipolysis of TG stores and efflux of fatty acids into the bloodstream, augmenting the problem. The presence of high levels of non-esterified fatty acids (NEFAs) in the bloodstream is proposed to function as a key mechanistic link between obesity and insulin resistance, type 2 diabetes, and metabolic dyslipidemia. Eventually, these NEFAs may be taken up ectopically by non-adipose tissues such as the liver and skeletal muscle, where they may be stored as TG or diacylglycerol and interfere with metabolic pathways such as the response to insulin, contributing to insulin resistance and the metabolic syndrome [58].

Differences exist in the metabolic properties of the various sites of adipose tissue. Visceral or abdominal fat stores are believed to pose a greater risk for the development of insulin resistance and the metabolic syndrome than subcutaneous fat stores. Reasons for this include reduced responsiveness of visceral fat to the anti-lipolytic effects of insulin (due to lower expression and activity of hormone sensitive lipase [HSL], reduced tyrosine phosphorylation of the insulin receptor, decreased insulin receptor substrate [IRS]-1 expression, and increased protein tyrosine phosphatase [PTP]-1B activity); greater responsiveness of visceral fat to the lipolysis-inducing effects of catecholamines; and decreased uptake and acylation of fatty acids compared with subcutaneous fat, all of which result in amplification of NEFA levels in the blood [59]. Visceral fat is also located conveniently for these NEFAs to enter portal circulation for direct delivery to the liver, where they pose risks to hepatic insulin responsiveness. Fructose consumption can induce perturbations in cell signaling and inflammatory cascades in insulin-sensitive tissues. In particular, the roles of cellular signaling molecules including nuclear factor kappa B (NFkB), tumor necrosis factor alpha (TNF-alpha), c-Jun amino terminal kinas 1 (JNK-1), protein tyrosine phosphatase 1B (PTP-1B), phosphatase and tensin homolog deleted on chromosome ten (PTEN), liver X receptor (LXR), farnesoid X receptor (FXR), and sterol regulatory element-binding protein-1c (SREBP-1c [60]. The contribution of fructose/sucrose in dyslipidemia was discussed above. Consuming such large amounts of fructose/sucrose can lead to development of a complete metabolic syndrome by increasing plasma TGs and altering hepatic glucose homeostasis, gaining weight, and decreasing insulin sensitivity. The triglyceride response to fructose ingestion appears to depend on whether or not a person is carbohydrate sensitive or insulin resistant. In one study, a diet containing 20 percent of energy as fructose significantly increased plasma triglyceride levels in male volunteers after five weeks, compared with a similar diet containing 20 percent of calories as cornstarch. The effect of the diet on triglyceride levels was more pronounced in hyperinsulinemic men (+66.7%) than in non-hyperinsulinemic men (+12.5%) [61].

Fructose and Uric Acid

Fructose consumption has been shown to increase serum uric acid levels. In a study of 21 male volunteers (ages 23-64 years), a diet containing 20 percent of energy as fructose (consumed for five weeks) significantly increased the mean serum uric acid concentration, compared with a similar diet containing 20 percent of energy as starch.[61-62] In another study of 11 healthy volunteers, diets containing 24 percent of carbohydrate as fructose did not alter serum uric acid levels when compared with a diet containing 24 percent of carbohydrate as sucrose.[63] However, as sucrose consists of 50-percent fructose, and as it has itself been shown to increase serum uric acid levels,[64] it is not an ideal control for evaluating the short-term metabolic effects of fructose. In addition to being a risk factor for gout, elevated uric acid levels are associated with an increased risk of cardiovascular disease. [65].

Fructose, Advanced Glycation End-Products, and Aging

Reducing sugars, such as fructose and glucose, react with proteins and amino acids to form substituted amino sugars. This reaction, known as the Maillard reaction (also called glycosylation or glycation), usually occurs at the site of a lysine side-chain. The initial products of the Maillard reaction undergo further reactions and rearrangements to form AGEs, which accumulate indefinitely on long-lived molecules such as collagen and DNA. There is evidence that AGEs play a role in the aging process;[66] in the pathogenesis of the vascular, renal, and ocular complications of diabetes;[67-69] and in the development of atherosclerosis.[70,71] fructose is much more reactive than glucose with respect to participation in glycosylation reactions. *In vitro*, the rate of non-enzymatic glycosylation of hemoglobin was 7.5 times greater,[72] and the rate of protein cross-linking (a manifestation of aging) was 10 times greater,[73] in the presence of fructose than in the presence of glucose. Thus, the large percentage increases in serum fructose concentrations that occur after ingestion of fructose or sucrose may have clinical consequences, even though absolute fructose concentrations remain low in comparison with glucose concentrations. Rats were fed a commercial diet for one year and had free access to water or to solutions containing 250 g/L of fructose, glucose, or sucrose. [74]None of the sugar solutions had any effect on plasma glucose concentrations. However, glycosylated hemoglobin levels and concentrations of lipid peroxidation products were significantly higher in fructose-fed rats than in those given sucrose, glucose, or water. In addition, three measures of aging – the solubility, cross-linking, and fluorescence of collagen – were each significantly greater in the fructose group than in the other groups. These findings suggest that long-term fructose consumption may accelerate the aging process. The use of fructose in cooking also has the potential to cause adverse effects. AGEs form during the heating of common foods and, in contrast to *in vivo* AGE formation, they can develop during cooking much more rapidly and in far greater concentrations.[75] Approximately 10 percent of ingested AGEs are absorbed, of which two-thirds are retained in tissues in reactive forms.[75] Dietary AGEs have been shown to accelerate the progression of nephropathy and to shorten survival times in an animal model of diabetes.[76] In humans with diabetes, the mean concentration of C-reactive protein was 135-percent higher when the diet was high in AGEs than when cooking methods were altered to reduce the dietary AGE content.[75,76] The rate of AGE formation during cooking would presumebly be far greater in the presence of fructose than in the presence of a non-reducing sugar such as sucrose. While most of the AGE content of a typical Western diet is derived from the heating of high-protein or high-fat foods, such as meats, butter, and cheese,[77] the use of HFCS in the baking of breads, pastries, pies, and other foods would be expected to increase dietary AGE levels further.

Functional Bowel Disturbances

Unlike glucose, which is completely absorbed in the intestine, the capacity to absorb fructose is limited. Unabsorbed fructose may serve as an osmotic load that draws fluid into the intestinal lumen, resulting in symptoms such as diarrhea, abdominal pain, bloating, flatus, belching, and discomfort. Symptoms may also result from the action of colonic bacteria on unabsorbed fructose.[78] Approximately 50 percent of fructose malabsorbers experience gastrointestinal symptoms after ingesting fructose.[79] In a study of 183 patients with unexplained gastrointestinal symptoms who were challenged with 50 g of fructose, 73 percent showed evidence of fructose malabsorption [80]. In patients with gastrointestinal symptoms and fructose malabsorption, a diet free of, or low in, fructose often relieved symptoms.[79,81,82] Glucose enhances the absorption of fructose, and malabsorption of fructose typically occurs only if more fructose than glucose is present.[83] Thus, a person who malabsorbs fructose would usually show normal absorption of the same amount of fructose when administered as sucrose (which is 50% glucose) or as a mixture of equal parts glucose and fructose. [83] In contrast, sorbitol inhibits the absorption of fructose. Simultaneous ingestion of these two sugars in amounts, which by themselves are well tolerated, may elicit symptoms in some people.[84] HFCS, which contains more fructose than glucose, may be an important cause of symptoms in some patients with irritable bowel syndrome or other functional bowel disturbances.

CONCLUSION

The consumption of excessive amounts of sucrose, fructose or HFCS can lead to a wide range of health problems. Sweeteners use has increased considerably around the world and Soft drink beverage seems to be a major contributor for obesity, diabetes mellitus, hyperlipidemia, insulin resistance, hypertension, metabolic syndrome, and cardiovascular disease. In some respects, fructose and HFCS are probably even more dangerous than sucrose. Although there are still many gaps in our knowledge, a prudent approach would be to keep the intake of these sweeteners to a minimum.

REFERENCES

[1] Elliott, S. S., Keim, N. L., Stern, J. S. et al. Fructose, weight gain, and the insulin resistance syndrome. *Am. J. Clin. Nutr.* 2002;76:911-922.

[2] Bantle, J. P., Laine, D. C., Thomas, J. W. Metabolic effects of dietary fructose and sucrose in types I and II diabetic subjects. *JAMA* 1986;256:3241-3246.

[3] Nseir, W., Nassar, F., Assy, N. Soft drinks consumption and nonalcoholic fatty liver disease. *World J. Gastroenterol.* 2010 ; 16: 2579-2588

[4] Cook, G. C. Absorption products of D(-) fructose in man. *Clin. Sci.* 1969;37:675-687

[5] Dencker, H., Meeuwisse, G., Norryd, C., Olin, T., Tranberg, K. G. Intestinal transport of carbohydrates as measured by portal catheterization in man. *Digestion.* 1973;9:514-524

[6] Macdonald, I., Keyser, A., Pacy, D. Some effects, in man, of varying the load of glucose, sucrose, fructose, or sorbitol on various metabolites in blood. *Am. J. Clin. Nutr.* 1978;31:1305-1311

[7] Mayes, P. A . Intermediary metabolism of fructose. American *Journal of Clinical Nutritio. 1993; 5: 754S (12)*

[8] Sanyal, A. J., Campbell-Sargent, C., Mirshahi, F., Rizzo, W. B., Contos, M. J., Sterling, R. K., Luketic, V. A., Shiffman, M. L., Clore, J. N. Nonalcoholic steatohepatitis: association of insulin resistance and mitochondrial abnormalities. *Gastroenterology* 2001; 120: 1183-1192

[9] Teff, K. L., Elliott, S. S., Tschöp, M., Kieffer, T. J., Rader, D., Heiman, M., Townsend, R. R., Keim, N. L., D'Alessio, D., Havel, P. J. Dietary fructose reduces circulating insulin and leptin, attenuates postprandial suppression of ghrelin, and increases triglycerides in women. *J. Clin. Endocrinol. Metab.* 2004; 89: 2963-2972

[10] Teff, K. L., Grudziak, J., Townsend, R. R., Dunn, T. N., Grant, R. W., Adams, S. H., Keim, N. L., Cummings, B. P., Stanhope, K. L., Havel, P. J. Endocrine and metabolic effects of consuming fructose- and glucose-sweetened beverages with meals in obese men and women: influence of insulin resistance on plasma triglyceride responses. *J. Clin. Endocrinol. Metab.* 2009; 94: 1562-1569

[11] Samuel, V. T. Fructose induced lipogenesis: from sugar to fat to insulin resistance. *Trends Endocrinol. Metab.* 2011 ;22:60-5.

[12] Matsuzaka, T., Shimano, H., Yahagi, N., Amemiya-Kudo, M., Okazaki, H., Tamura, Y.,Iizuka, Y., Ohashi, K., Tomita, S., Sekiya, M., Hasty, A., Nakagawa, Y., Sone, H., Toyoshima, H., Ishibashi, S., Osuga, J., Yamada, N. Insulin-independent induction of sterol regulatory element-binding protein-1c expression in the livers of streptozotocin-treated mice. *Diabetes* 2004; 53: 560-569

[13] Nagai, Y., Nishio, Y., Nakamura, T., Maegawa, H., Kikkawa, R., Kashiwagi A. Amelioration of high fructose-induced metabolic derangements by activation of PPARalpha. *Am. J. Physiol. Endocrinol. Metab.* 2002; 282: E1180-E1190

[14] Stanhope, K. L., Schwarz, J. M., Keim, N. L., Griffen, S. C., Bremer, A. A., Graham, J. L., Hatcher, B., Cox, C. L., Dyachenko, A., Zhang, W., McGahan, J. P., Seibert, A., Krauss, R. M., Chiu, S., Schaefer, E. J., Ai, M., Otokozawa, S., Nakajima, K., Nakano, T., Beysen, C., Hellerstein, M. K., Berglund, L., Havel, P. J. Consuming fructose-sweetened, not glucose-sweetened, beverages increases visceral adiposity and lipids and decreases insulin sensitivity in overweight/obese humans. *J. Clin. Invest.* 2009; 119: 1322-1334

[15] McDevitt, R. M., Bott, S. J., Harding, M., Coward, W. A., Bluck, L. J., Prentice, A. M. De novo lipogenesis during controlled overfeeding with sucrose or glucose in lean and obese women. *Am. J. Clin. Nutr.* 2001; 74: 737-746

[16] Zelber-Sagi, S., Nitzan-Kaluski, D., Goldsmith, R., Webb, M., Blendis, L., Halpern, Z., Oren, R. Long term nutritional intake and the risk for non-alcoholic fatty liver disease(NAFLD): a population based study. *J. Hepatol.* 2007; 47: 711-717

[17] Cusi, K. Nonalcoholic fatty liver disease in type 2 diabetes mellitus. *Curr. Opin. Endocrinol. Diabetes. Obes.* 2009; 16: 141-149

[18] Blakely, S. R., Hallfrisch, J., Reiser, S., Prather, E. S. Long-term effects of moderate fructose feeding on glucose tolerance parameters in rats. *J. Nutr.* 1981; 111: 307-314

[19] Thorburn, A. W., Crapo, P. A., Griver, K., Wallace, P., Henry, R. R. Long-term effects of dietary fructose on carbohydrate metabolism in non-insulin-dependent diabetes mellitus. *Metabolism* 1990; 39: 58-63

[20] Cohen, A. M., Teitelbaum, A., Rosenman, E. Diabetes induced by a high fructose diet. *Metabolism* 1977; 26: 17-24

[21] Schulze, M. B., Manson, J. E., Ludwig, D. S., Colditz, G. A., Stampfer, M. J., Willett, W. C., Hu, F. B. Sugar-sweetened beverages, weight gain, and incidence of type 2 diabetes in young and middle-aged women. *JAMA* 2004; 292: 927-934

[22] Ludwig, D. S., Peterson, K. E., Gortmaker, S. L. Relation between consumption of sugar-sweetened drinks and childhood obesity: a prospective, observational analysis. *Lancet* 2001; 357: 505-508

[23] Allen, R. J., Brook, M., Lister, R. E., Sim, A. K., Warwick, M. H. Metabolic differences between dietary liquid glucose and sucrose. *Nature* 1966; 211: 1104

[24] Nagata, R., Nishio, Y., Sekine, O., Nagai, Y., Maeno, Y., Ugi, S., Maegawa, H., Kashiwagi, A. Single nucleotide polymorphism (-468 Gly to A) at the promoter region of SREBP-1c associates with genetic defect of fructose-induced hepatic lipogenesis [corrected]. *J. Biol. Chem.* 2004; 279: 29031-29042

[25] Waxman, A. WHO global strategy on diet, physical activity and health. *Food Nutr. Bull.* 2004; 25: 292-302

[26] Willms, J. D., Tremblay, M. S., Katzmarzyk, P. T. Geographic and demographic variation in the prevalence of overweight Canadian children. *Obes. Res.* 2003; 11: 668-673

[27] Dubois, L., Farmer, A., Girard, M., Peterson, K. Regular sugar-sweetened beverage consumption between meals increases risk of overweight among preschool-aged children. *J. Am. Diet Assoc.* 2007; 107: 924-934; discussion 934-935

[28] James, J., Thomas, P., Cavan, D., Kerr, D. Preventing childhood obesity by reducing consumption of carbonated drinks: cluster randomised controlled trial. *BMJ* 2004; 328: 1237

[29] Assy, N., Nasser, G., Kamayse, I., Nseir, W., Beniashvili, Z., Djibre, A., Grosovski, M. Soft drink consumption linked with fatty liver in the absence of traditional risk factors. *Can. J. Gastroenterol.* 2008; 22: 811-816

[30] Abid, A., Taha, O., Nseir, W., Farah, R., Grosovski, M., Assy, N. Soft drink consumption is associated with fatty liver disease independent of metabolic syndrome. *J. Hepatol.* 2009; 51: 918-924

[31] Tuovinen, C. G., Bender, A. E. Some metabolic effects of prolonged feeding of starch, sucrose, fructose and carbohydrate-free diet in the rat. *Nutr. Metab.* 1975; 19: 161-172

[32] Davail, S., Rideau, N., Bernadet, M. D., André, J. M., Guy, G., Hoo-Paris, R. Effects of dietary fructose on liver steatosis in overfed mule ducks. *Horm. Metab. Res.* 2005; 37: 32-35

[33] Nandhini, A. T., Balakrishnan, S. D., Anuradha, C. V. Response of liver antioxidant system to taurine in rats fed high fructose diet. *Indian J. Exp. Biol.* 2002; 40: 1016-1019

[34] Kelley, G. L., Allan, G., Azhar, S. High dietary fructose induces a hepatic stress response resulting in cholesterol and lipid dysregulation. *Endocrinology* 2004; 145: 548-555

[35] Wolfe, B. M., Ahuja, S. P., Marliss, E. B. Effects of intravenously administered fructose and glucose on splanchnic amino acid and carbohydrate metabolism in hypertriglyceridemic men. *J. Clin. Invest.* 1975; 56: 970-977

[36] Ackerman, Z., Oron-Herman, M., Grozovski, M., Rosenthal, T., Pappo, O., Link, G., Sela, B. A. Fructose-induced fatty liver disease: hepatic effects of blood pressure and plasma triglyceride reduction. *Hypertension* 2005; 45: 1012-1018

[37] Porikos, K. P., Van Itallie, T. B. Diet-induced changes in serum transaminase and triglyceride levels in healthy adult men. Role of sucrose and excess calories. *Am. J. Med.* 1983; 75: 624-630

[38] Howard, B. V., Wylie-Rosett, J. Sugar and cardiovascular disease: A statement for healthcare professionals from the Committee on Nutrition of the Council on Nutrition, Physical Activity, and Metabolism of the American Heart Association. *Circulation* 2002; 106: 523-527

[39] Havel, P. J. Dietary fructose: implications for dysregulation of energy homeostasis and lipid/carbohydrate metabolism. *Nutr. Rev.* 2005; 63: 133-157

[40] Taghibiglou, C., Carpentier, A., Van Iderstine, S. C., Chen, B., Rudy, D., Aiton, A., Lewis, G. F., Adeli, K. Mechanisms of hepatic very low density lipoprotein overproduction in insulin resistance. Evidence for enhanced lipoprotein assembly, reduced intracellular ApoB degradation, and increased microsomal triglyceride transfer protein in a fructose-fed hamster model. *J. Biol. Chem.* 2000; 275: 8416-8425

[41] Taghibiglou, C., Rashid-Kolvear, F., Van Iderstine, S. C., Le-Tien, H, Fantus, I. G., Lewis, G. F., Adeli, K. Hepatic very low density lipoprotein-ApoB overproduction is associated with attenuated hepatic insulin signaling and overexpression of protein-tyrosine phosphatase 1B in a fructose-fed hamster model of insulin resistance. *J. Biol. Chem.* 2002; 277: 793-803

[42] Bode, J. C., Zelder, O., Rumpelt, H. J., Wittkamp, U. Depletion of liver adenosine phosphates and metabolic effects of intravenous infusion of fructose or sorbitol in man and in the rat. *Eur. J. Clin. Invest.* 1973; 3: 436-441

[43] Oberhaensli, R. D., Galloway, G. J., Taylor, D. J., Bore, P. J., Radda, G. K. Assessment of human liver metabolism by phosphorus-31 magnetic resonance spectroscopy. *Br. J. Radiol.* 1986; 59: 695-699

[44] Cortez-Pinto, H., Chatham, J., Chacko, V. P., Arnold, C., Rashid, A., Diehl, A. M. Alterations in liver ATP homeostasis in human nonalcoholic steatohepatitis: a pilot study. *JAMA* 1999; 282: 1659-1664

[45] Adachi, F., Yu, D. T., Phillips, M. J. An ultrastructural study of fructose-induced hepatic cell injury. Comparison of human and experimental lesions. *Virchows Arch. B Cell Pathol.* 1972; 10: 200-209

[46] Cirillo, P., Sautin, Y. Y., Kanellis, J., Kang, D. H., Gesualdo, L., Nakagawa, T., Johnson, R. J. Systemic inflammation, metabolic syndrome and progressive renal disease. *Nephrol. Dial. Transplant.* 2009; 24: 1384-1387

[47] Ouyang, X., Cirillo, P., Sautin, Y., McCall, S., Bruchette, J. L., Diehl, A. M., Johnson, R. J., Abdelmalek, M. F. Fructose consumption as a risk factor for non-alcoholic fatty liver disease. *J. Hepatol.* 2008; 48: 993-999

[48] Burant, C. F., Saxena, M. Rapid reversible substrate regulation of fructose transporter expression in rat small intestine and kidney. *Am. J. Physiol.* 1994; 267: G71-G79

[49] Korieh, A., Crouzoulon, G. Dietary regulation of fructose metabolism in the intestine and in the liver of the rat. Duration of the effects of a high fructose diet after the return to the standard diet. *Arch. Int. Physiol. Biochim. Biophys.* 1991; 99: 455-460

[50] Stirpe, F., Della Corte, E., Bonetti, E., Abbondanza, A., Abbati, A., De Stefano, F. Fructose-induced hyperuricaemia. *Lancet* 1970; 2: 1310-1311

[51] Israel, K. D., Michaelis, O. E. 4th, Reiser, S., Keeney, M. Serum uric acid, inorganic phosphorus, and glutamic-oxalacetic transaminase and blood pressure in carbohydrate-sensitive adults consuming three different levels of sucrose. *Ann. Nutr. Metab.* 1983; 27: 425-435

[52] Sartorio, A., Del Col, A., Agosti, F., Mazzilli, G., Bellentani, S., Tiribelli, C., Bedogni, G. Predictors of non-alcoholic fatty liver disease in obese children. *Eur. J. Clin. Nutr.* 2007; 61: 877-883

[53] Nakagawa, T., Hu, H., Zharikov, S., Tuttle, K. R., Short, R. A., Glushakova, O., Ouyang, X., Feig, D. I., Block, E. R., Herrera-Acosta, J., Patel, J. M., Johnson, R. J. A causal role for uric acid in fructose-induced metabolic syndrome. *Am. J. Physiol. Renal. Physiol.* 2006; 290: F625-F631

[54] Khosla, U. M., Zharikov, S., Finch, J. L., Nakagawa, T., Roncal, C., Mu, W., Krotova, K., Block, E. R., Prabhakar, S., Johnson, R. J. Hyperuricemia induces endothelial dysfunction. *Kidney Int.* 2005; 67: 1739-1742

[55] Reaven, G. M. Banting lecture 1988. Role of insulin resistance in human disease. *Diabetes* 1988;37:1595-1607

[56] National Cholesterol Education Program (NCEP) Expert Panel on Detection, Evaluation, and Treatment of High Blood Cholesterol in Adults (Adult Treatment Panel III). Third Report of the National Cholesterol Education Program (NCEP) Expert Panel on Detection, Evaluation, and Treatment of High Blood Cholesterol in Adults (Adult Treatment Panel III) final report. *Circulation* 2002;106:3143-3421

[57] Alberti, K. G., Eckel, R. H., Grundy, S. M., Zimmet, P. Z., Cleeman, J. I., Donato, K. A., Fruchart, J. C., James, W. P., Loria, C. M., Smith, S. C. Jr.; International Diabetes Federation Task Force on Epidemiology and Prevention; Hational Heart, Lung, and Blood Institute; American Heart Association; World Heart Federation; International Atherosclerosis Society; International Association for the Study of Obesity. Harmonizing the metabolic syndrome: a joint interim statement of the International Diabetes Federation Task Force on Epidemiology and Prevention; National Heart, Lung, and Blood Institute; American Heart Association; World Heart Federation; International Atherosclerosis Society; and International Association for the Study of Obesity. *Circulation*. 2009 ;120:1640-5.

[58] Hansen, E., Hajri, T., Abumrad, N. N. Is all fat the same? The role of fat in the pathogenesis of the metabolic syndrome and type 2 diabetes mellitus. *Surgery* 2006;139:711-76

[59] Reynisdottir, S., Dauzats, M., Thörne, A., Langin, D. Comparison of hormone-sensitive lipase activity in visceral and subcutaneous human adipose tissue. *J. Clin. Endocrinol. Metab.*1997;82:4162-4166

[60] Rutledge, A. C., Adeli, K. Fructose and the metabolic syndrome: pathophysiology and molecular mechanisms. *Nutr. Rev.* 2007;65:S13-23 61.

[61] Reiser, S., Powell, A. S., Scholfield, D. J. et al. Blood lipids, lipoproteins, apoproteins, and uric acid in men fed diets containing fructose or high-amylose cornstarch. *Am. J. Clin. Nutr.* 1989;49:832-839.

[62] Emmerson, B. T. Effect of oral fructose on urate production. *Ann. Rheum. Dis.* 1974;33:276-280.

[63] Crapo, P. A., Kolterman, O. G. The metabolic effects of 2-week fructose feeding in normal subjects. *Am. J. Clin. Nutr.* 1984;39:525-534.

[64] Kelsay, J. L., Behall, K. M., Moser, P. B., Prather, E. S. The effect of kind of carbohydrate in the diet and use of oral contraceptives on metabolism of young women. I. Blood and urinary lactate, uric acid, and phosphorus. *Am. J. Clin. Nutr.* 1977;30:2016-2022.

[65] Fang, J., Alderman, M. H. Serum uric acid and cardiovascular mortality the NHANES I. *epidemiologic follow-up study*, 1971-1992.

[66] Dills, W. L. Jr. Protein fructosylation: fructose and the Maillard reaction. *Am. J. Clin. Nutr.* 1993;58:779S-787S.

[67] Brownlee, M. Glycosylation products as toxic mediators of diabetic complications. *Annu. Rev. Med.* 1991;42:159-166.

[68] Howard, B. V., Wylie-Rosett, J. Sugar and cardiovascular disease: a statement for healthcare professionals from the Committee on Nutrition of the Council on Nutrition, Physical Activity, and Metabolism of the American Heart Association.*Circulation* 2002;106:523-527.

[69] Devamanoharan, P. S., Ali, A. H., Varma, S. D. Prevention of lens protein glycation by taurine. *Mol. Cell Biochem.* 1997;177:245-250.

[70] Lin, Y. T., Tseng, Y. Z., Chang, K. C. Aminoguanidine prevents fructose-induced arterial stiffening in Wistar rats: aortic impedance analysis. *Exp. Biol. Med. (Maywood)* 2004;229:1038-1045.

[71] Cerami, A., Vlassara, H., Brownlee, M. Protein glycosylation and the pathogenesis ofatherosclerosis. *Metabolism* 1985;34:37-42.

[72] Bunn, H. F., Higgins, P. J. Reaction of monosaccharides with proteins: possible evolutionary significance. *Science* 1981;213:222-224.

[73] McPherson, J. D., Shilton, B. H., Walton, D. J. Role of fructose in glycation and cross-linking of proteins. *Biochemistry* 1988;27:1901-1907.

[74] Levi, B., Werman, M. J. Long-term fructose consumption accelerates glycation and several age-related variables in male rats. *J. Nutr.* 1998;128:1442-1449.

[75] Vlassara, H., Cai, W., Crandall, J. et al. Inflammatory mediators are induced by dietary glycotoxins, a major risk factor for diabetic angiopathy. *Proc. Natl. Acad. Sci. U S A* 2002;99:15596-15601.

[76] Zheng, F., He, C., Cai, W. et al. Prevention of diabetic nephropathy in mice by a diet low in glycoxidation products. *Diabetes Metab. Res. Rev.* 2002;18:224-237.

[77] Goldberg, T., Cai, W., Peppa, M. et al. Advanced glycoxidation end products in commonly consumed foods. *J. Am. Diet Assoc.* 2004;104:1287-1291.

[78] Born, P., Zech, J., Lehn, H. et al. Colonic bacterial activity determines the symptoms in people with fructose-malabsorption. *Hepatogastroenterology* 1995;42:778-785.

[79] Ledochowski, M., Widner, B., Bair, H. et al.Fructose- and sorbitol-reduced diet improves mood and gastrointestinal disturbances in fructose malabsorbers. *Scand. J. Gastroenterol.* 2000;35:1048-1052.

[80] Rumessen, J. J., Gudmand-Hoyer, E. Functional bowel disease: malabsorption and abdominal distress after ingestion of fructose, sorbitol, and fructose-sorbitol mixtures. *Gastroenterology* 1988;95:694-700.

[81] Andersson, D. E., Nygren, A. Four cases of longstanding diarrhoea and colic pains cured by fructose-free diet – a pathogenetic discussion. *Acta. Med. Scand.* 1978;203:87-92.

[82] Fernandez-Banares, F., Esteve-Pardo, M., De Leon, R. et al. Sugar malabsorption in functional bowel disease: clinical implications. *Am. J. Gastroenterol.* 1993;88:2044-2050.

[83] Ament, M. E. Malabsorption of apple juice and pear nectar in infants and children: clinical implications. *J. Am. Coll. Nutr.* 1996;15:26S-29S.

[84] Rumessen, J. J., Gudmand-Hoyer, E. Malabsorption of fructose-sorbitol mixtures. Interactions causing abdominal distress. *Scand. J. Gastroenterol.* 1987;22:431-436.

In: Fructose
Editors: Brandon M. Johnston and Aaron B. Collins
ISBN: 978-1-62081-126-9

Chapter 6

FRUCTOSE FACILITATES ALCOHOL METABOLISM

I. Onyesom[*]
Department of Medical Biochemistry,
Delta State University, Abraka, Nigeria.

DEFINITION, DISCOVERY AND PROBLEMS OF ALCOHOL

Alcohol is a clear, colourless, mobile, volatile, inflammable liquid with a characteristic spirituous, faint, sharp odour of burning taste formed by vinous fermentation. Chemically, alcohols are a group of organic compounds with hydroxyl (-OH) group attached to a hydrocarbon (R-) chain, generally represented as R-OH. The OH group determines the behaviour of alcohols. The alcohol contained in various alcoholic beverages (wine, beer, gin, whiskey, and spirits) is ethanol (C_2H_5OH), a small molecular weight, non-polar compound which does not require modification or digestion before absorption.

Ethanol was probably discovered accidentally in the pre-agricultural gathering stage, and early men presumably liked the euphorigenic effect, if not the taste, and so, proceeded to purposeful production. Some anthropologists have suggested that early Stone Age agricultural settlements arose from a need to make wine rather than grow food. Since discovered, ethanol has continued to play various roles in the history of mankind, and in most cases, alcohol use (consumption) has been abused leading to problems.

The abuse of alcohol consumption causes alcoholism, and this disease has remained difficult to define, but WHO (1952) provided a frequently quoted definition. The definition appears long and sometimes confusing. A concise definition was suggested by Davies (1973). He defined alcoholism as "*the intermittent or continual ingestion of alcohol leading to dependency or harm*". Alcoholism constitutes major problems in both the Western World and developing countries, yet only recently that the reasons why an individual should develop alcohol-related problems, injury or dependence are becoming understood. A complex of social, psychiatric, psychological and biochemical factors may interact to predispose an individual to alcoholism. Alcoholism is a preventable disease of choice, hence largely

[*] e-mail: onyesominno@yahoo.co.uk

neglected, yet it constitutes great burden and menace to society. At present however, the need to search for agents that can stimulate the elimination of alcohol from blood stream and reverse its effects in the body is vigorously being pursued. Fructose has been observed to stimulate the clearance of alcohol from bloodstream in both human and animal experiments conducted independently at different times and places. This review therefore attempts to provide a highlight of research frontiers in this field of study.

ALCOHOL PHARMACOKINETICS

Absorption: When consumed, alcohol is absorbed from all parts of the gastrointestinal tract, GIT, mainly by simple diffusion into the blood without digestion or modification. In a fasting subject, about 20% to 25% and 75% to 80% of a dose of alcohol is absorbed from the stomach and small intestine, respectively. But if the stomach is full, as much as 70% of ingested alcohol can be absorbed from the stomach (Cortot, *et al.*, 1986).

Distribution: Absorbed alcohol is distributed mainly in the body water due to low solubility in lipids. It is therefore, found in body tissues and fluids including sweat, urine, breath, cerebrospinal fluid (CSF), synovial fluid (CF), inasmuch as they contain water. The overall distribution volume is approximately 0.73L/kg body weight for males and 0.59L/kg body weight for females. The gender difference is due to the lower water content in females, and as a consequence higher ethanol levels are found in females than in males after the intake of a standard amount of alcohol per body weight (NIAAA, 1997).

Elimination: About 90% to 98% of ingested alcohol is eliminated from the body through oxidative metabolism in the liver, and the remaining 2% to 10% is eliminated unchanged through excretion in breath, sweat, faeces, milk and saliva. However, minute amounts are conjugated with glucuronic or sulphuric acids, and excreted in urine.

The Oxidative Metabolism of Ethanol

The basic pathways of alcohol oxidative metabolism involve the progressive oxidation of ethanol to acetaldehyde, and then, to acetate. The major site of this oxidation is the liver parenchymal cells, but other potential sites include GIT (first-pass metabolism), vascular tissue and brain.

The hepatocyte (liver cell) contains three main pathways for ethanol oxidative metabolism, each located in a different subcellular compartment. The alcohol dehydrogenase, ADH pathway of the cytosol or the soluble fraction of the cell, the microsomal ethanol oxidizing system, MEOS, located in the endoplasmic reticulum, and catalase located in the peroxisomes (Lieber, 1991). These three distinct pathways result in the production of acetaldehyde, a highly toxic metabolite which has potent vasoactive properties. It has been implicated in alcohol dependency via the formation of opioid-like insoquinolines, and tissue damage through the formation of reactive oxygen species, ROS, acetaldehyde adducts and immunological reactions.

The further oxidation of acetaldehyde to acetate is catalyzed by acetaldehyde dehydrogenase, ALDH, the predominantly low K_m mitochondrial enzyme. Some of the acetate produced by the action of ALDH is converted to acetylCoA in the liver and oxidized or converted to amino acids, fatty acids, or glycogen in the same way as acetylCoA from other sources. However, large amounts of acetate pass into the systemic circulation and are taken up in other tissues, converted to acetylCoA, and oxidized to carbon (IV) oxide and water via the Kreb's cycle.

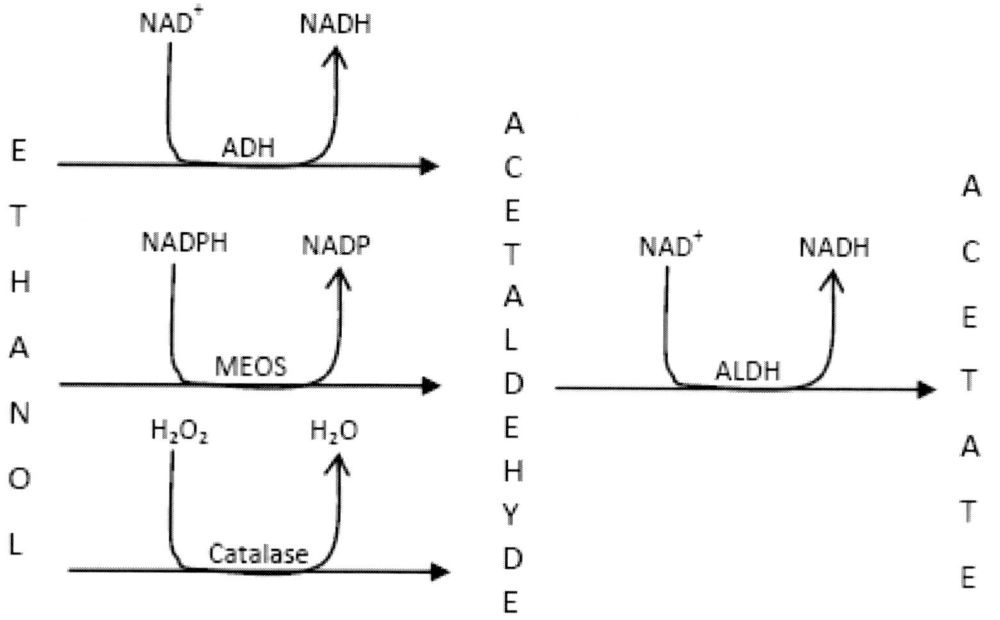

Figure 1. Principal pathways of ethanol oxidation (Peters and Preedy, 1998).

The rate-limiting step in the whole oxidative metabolism of alcohol is the ADH step. In well nourished individuals, the rate is determined 70% by the concentration of the ADH enzyme and 30% by the NAD^+ concentration or NAD^+: NADH ratio (Kalant and Khanna, 1987). Non – Oxidative Metabolism of Alcohol: The capacity of alcohol to form ethyl esters e.g. fatty acid ethyl esters, FAEE *in vivo* has been reported (Godman and Deykin, 1963) and this contributes to the metabolism of ingested alcohol, though FAEE has been observed (Laposata and Lange, 1986; Bora, *et al.*, 1996) to play a role in the production of alcohol – induced injury especially in organs that lack oxidative alcohol metabolism.

In several isolated studies, the metabolism of ethanol has been associated with increase in blood lactate leading to secondary hyperuricaemia (Onyesom, 2003), increase in blood and hepatic lipids especially triacylglycerol (Lieber, 1992; Onyesom and Anosike, 2005). The effect of alcohol metabolism on blood glucose has remained controversial. Some have reported hypoglycaemia (Lieber, 1992), others hyperglycaemia (Lieber, 1997; Onyesom and Oriero, 2005). These observations are however influenced by dose, duration of intake and nutritional status of the subjects concerned.

The first step in the oxidation of alcohol generates an excess of reducing equivalents in the cytosol, primarily as NADH, with marked shift in the cytosolic redox potential, and this is the hallmark of the identified metabolic consequences of alcohol ingestion.

Biochemical Basis of the Metabolic Consequences of Alcohol

Urate: The increase in cytosolic NADH : NAD^+ ratio causes an increase in the lactate : pyruvate ratio (Figure 2) mediated via lactate dehydrogenase. The increase in lactate induces acidosis and reduces the capacity of the kidney to excrete urate, leading to secondary hyperuricaemia. The increased $NADH/NAD^+$ ratio in the mitochondria by ALDH increases the β-hydroxy butyrate/acetoacetate ratio with development of ketosis. The induced ketosis coupled with the enhanced purine breakdown may also promote the hyperuricaemia (Faller and Fox, 1982).

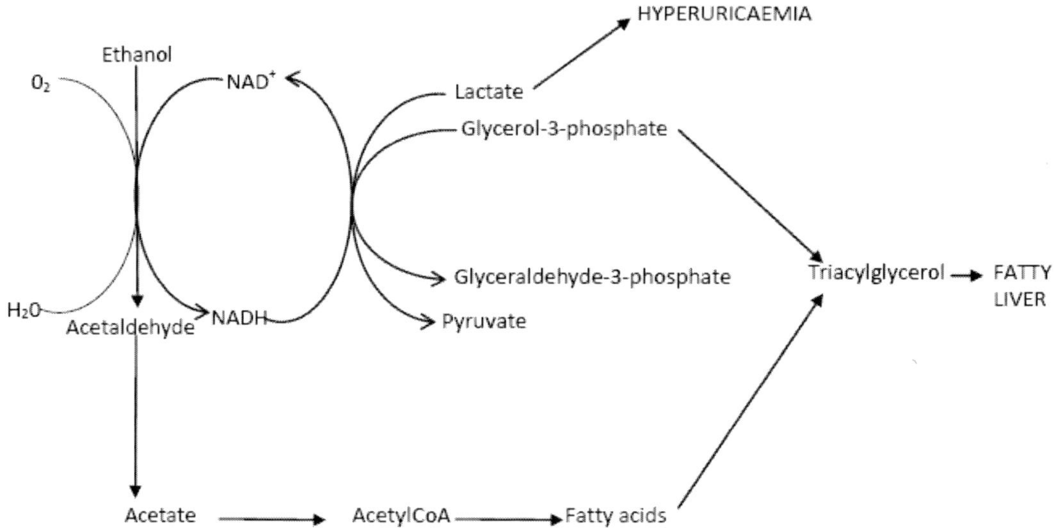

Figure 2. Some consequences of ethanol metabolism (Kalant and Khanna, 1987).

Lipids: The increased $NADH/NAD^+$ ratio raises the concentration of α-glycerophosphate which favours hepatic triacylglycerol accumulation by trapping fatty acids (Figure 2). In addition, excess NADH may promote fatty acid synthesis. Fatty acids of different sources can accumulate as triacylglycerol in the liver due to different metabolic disturbances which include enhanced hepatic lipogenesis, decreased hepatic release of lipoproteins, increased mobilization of peripheral fat, enhanced hepatic uptake of circulating lipids and, most importantly, decreased fatty acids oxidation, whether as a function of the reduced citric acid cycle activity secondary to the altered redox potential or as a consequence of permanent changes in mitochondrial structure and functions (Lieber, 1992).

HDL-cholesterol levels increase with moderate alcohol consumption, a tendency that has a cardioprotective effect (Lau, *et al.*, 1995). However, moderate alcohol intoxication occasionally causes severe hypoglycaemia (Lieber, 1992), due in part, to the block of hepatic gluconeogenesis by ethanol, again as a consequence of the increased $NADH/NAD^+$ ratio in subjects whose glycogen stores are already depleted by starvation or who have pre-existing abnormalities in carbohydrate metabolism, and this could result in sudden death. Paradoxically, hyperglycaemia indeed, may also occur in association with alcoholism. Its mechanism is still obscure, but glucose intolerance may be due, at least in part, to decreased peripheral glucose utilization (Lieber, 1997).

ALCOHOLISM AND RELATED PROBLEMS

Alcoholism is a primary, chronic disease with genetic, psychosocial, and environmental factors influencing its development and manifestations. The disease is often progressive and fatal. It is characterized by impaired control over drinking, pre-occupation with alcohol, use of alcohol despite adverse consequence, and distortions in thinking. Each of these symptoms may be continuous or periodic.

Clinical Presentations of Alcoholism

Liver: The liver being the major site of ethanol oxidation remains the primary target of ethanol toxicity. Alcohol-induced hepatic dysfunction as evidenced by biomarkers have been documented in animals (Onyesom and Anosike, 2007) and humans (Onyesom, *et al.*, 2007a). Microstructural alterations in hepatic lobules, an indication of liver damage by ethanol has been observed in experimental animals (Onyesom and Ekanem, 2011). It has been estimated that the minimum alcohol intake associated with appreciable liver damage is 16 units of alcohol daily for 5 years (Sherlock, 1995). Hepatocytes remain sensitive to alcohol for months after the cessation of heavy drinking.

Brain: The sedation produced by social drinking is accompanied by loss of inhibitory control of emotions, and the subjects become talkative and emotionally labile. Diminished fine motor skills, diminished cognition, peripheral motor/sensory neuropathy, impairment in sensory acuity causing altered sensation, motor ataxia and slurred speech, coupled with movement disorders have been reported (Neiman, *et al.*, 1990). In animals, alcohol administration alters brain glucose and lipids, and induced brain damage (Onyesom, *et al.*, 2007b). Data on alcohol consumption suggest that low levels of alcohol consumption, below 390g weekly, may have some protective effect on the cerebral vasculature, but heavy consumption, over 400g weekly predisposes to both hemorrhagic and non hemorrhagic stroke (Gill, *et al.*, 1991).

The most common manifestations of altered brain function of the alcoholics are the symptoms of inebriation, followed in frequency by the withdrawal syndromes of tremor, confusion, hallucinations, delirium tremens and convulsions. These are usually reversible functional changes.

Much less common but frequently irreversible changes are the metabolic disorders associated with protracted steady drinking and in most instances, nutritional deficiencies. These include: Wernicke-Korsakoff syndrome, peripheral neuropathy, cerebellar degeneration, cerebral degeneration, amblyopia, central pontine myelination of the corpus callosum (Marchiafava-Bignami disease).

Hypertension: Consumption of more than 2 units (between 20-24g) of ethanol a day results in a dose-dependent rise in blood pressure (Kei, *et al.*, 1993; Kaplan, 1995). In one study, it was demonstrated that the metabolism of blood acetaldehyde generated from ethanol caused increase in blood pressure in a manner that depends on its concentration (Onyesom and Naiho, 2005). The metabolism of acetaldehyde generates ROS known to oxidize NO, an important chemical regulator of blood pressure (Koppenol, 1998).

Pancreas: The association between alcohol and pancreatitis is at least as strong as the relationship between alcohol and liver disease. At postmortem examination, 18% to 47% of alcoholics dying of causes other than pancreatitis have some histological evidence of pancreatitis (Norton, *et al.*, 1998).

Alcohol is responsible for at least 30% and in some studies 60% to 90% of the cases of pancreatitis in the United States (Lopez, *et al.*, 1996). Although there is a wide range of individual variation, the average duration of alcohol consumption before the initial diagnosis of pancreatitis is 18 years in men and 11 years in women, suggesting that women have increased susceptibility.

Alcohol-induced stimulation of pancreatic juice, releases high protein concentration which can form plug upon precipitation. The plugs obstruct pancreatic ductules and cause calcific pancreatitis. Pancreatitis is characterized by elevation in amylase and lipase activities. Increased activities of salivary and serum (pancreatic) α-amylase have been reported among alcoholic subjects (Onyesom and Erude, 2004).

Pancreatic insufficiency could develop resulting in the destruction of insulin and glucagon-producing cells. When this occurs, the alcoholic develops diabetes mellitus and the need for insulin. Since glucagon level is also decreased, and too low to stimulate gluconeogenesis, these patients are brittle diabetics and are proned to hypoglycaemic attacks. This makes treatment cumbersome especially if alcohol consumption continues (Mendenhall and Weesner, 1989).

Heart: Chronic alcohol consumption produces alcoholic heart muscle disease, cardiomyopathy, a prevalent form of congestive heart failure. Several hypotheses have been proposed to explain this damaging effect but neither the mechanism nor ultimate toxin has been established (Liang, *et al.*, 1999), though Patel, *et al.* (1997) reported the features and possible mechanisms responsible for the development of alcoholic cardiomyopathy. The evidence suggests that the defects in myofibrillar protein turn-over occur in both acute and chronic alcohol studies.

Possible mechanisms to explain poor contractile function include alterations in cellular calcium, magnesium or phosphate homeostasis. The toxic effects of acetaldehyde or the formation of fatty acid ethyl esters, FAEE, may cause impairment of mitochondrial oxidative phosphorylation. Alternatively, reduced amounts of heat shock proteins, HSP, may result in poor assembly and interaction of proteins. Others include increase in HDL-cholesterol (Sesso and Gaziano, 1999), lower plasma fibrinogen and inhibited platelet aggregation (Pudedey, *et al.*, 1999).

Ethanol interferes with a number of myocardial metabolic steps and cellular mechanisms. A single key factor for the development of cardiac insufficiency can, however not be pointed out, although it is well known that ethanol interferes with lipid metabolism and fatty acid composition of sarcolemma as well as the properties of the membrane function of the sarcoplasmic reticulum (Waldenstrom, 1998). Chronic alcoholic patient has depressed cardiac output and ventricular hypocontractility (Moushmoush and Abi-Mansour, 1991).

Toxic substances such as cobalt chloride, foam stabilizer in beer (Knieriem and Herbertz, 1969), arsenic, in some wine drinks (Munzinge, 1987), lead, in some moonshiners (Asokan and Witham, 1972) may have been contributing factors affecting the development of cardiomyopathy in particular groups of chronic alcoholics. A controlled study suggests that susceptibility to alcoholic cardiomyopathy and myopathy appears to be more pronounced in women than in men (Urbano-Marquez, *et al.*, 1995).

Muscle: Alcoholic patients may develop proximal muscle weakness with elevated serum creatine kinase (CK) levels and myoglobinuria. Alcohol or its metabolite, acetaldehyde has been shown to affect sarcolemmal membranes with inhibition in ATP-dependent activity in a dose-dependent manner.

Alcohol causes both whole body and tissue –specific changes in protein metabolism due to increased nitrogen excretion with concomitant loss of lean tissue mass as well as loss of skeletal muscle protein (Preedy, *et al.*, 1999).

Treatment of Alcohol-Induced Problems

Obviously, extensive and prolonged ingestion of alcohol is injurious to health, but despite this, alcohol abuse and addiction are growing, and these constitute serious problems in many societies. The sociomedical damage and economic burden caused by alcohol is enormous, yet effective method (s) for ascertaining abuse and the mechanism of alcohol dependence are not well clarified. It suffices to add that till now, no single treatment can be claimed to be totally effective for combating the harmful effect of alcohol. Thus, treatment might theoretically be aimed at increasing the disappearance of alcohol from the body and counteracting its effects.

Many compounds have been tested for their claimed amethystic (anti-intoxicating) property. Recent example is the antiparkinsonian agent, amantadine, but the results are not very convincing. In serious intoxication with profound coma, CNS stimulants, analeptics, were occasionally used, but they are not very helpful because there is small margin between doses that are ineffective and those that are too large and cause seizures. Again, the benzodiazepine receptor inverse agonist, R_0 15 – 4513, can reverse some of the signs of alcohol intoxication, but it does not antagonize the lethal effect of ethanol overdose. The opioid antagonist, naloxone, has been reported to reverse alcoholic coma, but there are numerous reports that it has failed to work, and in experimental animals, it worked at does that produce analeptic effect. Supportive therapy (oral or intravenous administration of fluids) is being studied in order to discover substance(s) which could accelerate ethanol oxidation and provide a rapid means of clearing blood ethanol levels and reversing the effects of ethanol. Glucose and galactose (Kricka and Clark, 1979), sucrose and alanine (Rawat, 1974) were tested and found to have only minimal effect in reducing blood alcohol. Albeit, several results with fructose show that fructose administration significantly accelerated the clearance of alcohol from bloodstream and breath, making it a principal amethystic agent being studied.

Fructose Accelerates Blood Ethanol Elimination Rate (BEER)

The tendency of fructose to enhance blood ethanol elimination rate (BEER), the so-called 'fructose effect" was first observed by Carpenter and Lee (1937), and since then, the observation has been repeatedly confirmed (Stuhlfauth and Neumaier, 1951; Brown, *et al.*, 1972; Mascord *et al.*, 1991; Berman, *et al.*, 2003; Onyesom and Anosike, 2004).

Table 1 shows the changes in alcohol oxidokinetic data induced by oral fructose in man.

Oral fructose reduced the total duration of intoxication, that is, the time taken to reach zero BAL by 41.9% in the men and 40.0% in the women (Table 1).

Blood ethanol clearance rates in both the male and female subjects were increased by 66.1% and 92.6%, respectively, in the presence of fructose, and these increased rates were significant ($P<0.05$; Table 1). The gender differences in the oxidokinetic data have been attributed to the body water content.

Table 1. Changes in mean alcohol oxidokinetic data induced by oral fructose in man

Oxidokinetic parameter	Male (n=20)		Female (n=20)	
	Ethanol alone	Ethanol + Fructose	Ethanol alone	Ethanol + Fructose
Peak blood alcohol level, PBAL (mM)	20.2±0.5	16.5±0.5	20.9±1.0	21.0±0.7
Time to attain PBAL (min)	51.0±12.6	39.0±10.2	39.5±12.5	39.0±12.0
Time to reach zero BAL (min)	325±30	189±29	285±41	171±18
Blood alcohol clearance rate (mM/Min)	0.076± 0.011	0.127± 0.015	0.094± 0.011	0.181± 0.018

Onyesom and Anosike, Afr J. Drug Alcohol Stud. 3 (1and2):21-30; 2004.

The total body weight of men is composed of 55% to 65% water, while that of women is 45% to 55% water. Therefore, alcohol tends to be more diluted in the body of males than females. In previous reports, fructose has been observed to increase blood alcohol clearance by about 50% (Brown, et al., 1972), 80% (Rogers, et al., 1987; Mascord, et al., 1991) and 100% (Rawat, 1974). However, other workers have failed to confirm the "fructose effect" (Schmidt, et al., 1995).

Mechanisms of the Stimulatory Effect of Fructose on Blood Ethanol Elimination Rate (BEER)

The mechanism by which fructose accelerates alcohol metabolism is uncertain, but several interesting hypotheses have been proposed, and the most famous seems to be that, since the rate of alcohol oxidation by hepatic ADH is 30% dependent upon the rate of re-oxidation of NADH, the metabolism of fructose to sorbitol or to glycerol utilizes NADH and so, offers the means of re-oxidizing NADH. This facilitates further alcohol metabolism. Therefore, in the presence of alcohol, the metabolism of fructose in the liver is diverted from NAD^+ to NADH – requiring pathways, which in turn generate the NAD^+ needed for alcohol oxidation (Figure 3). Available evidence (Tygstrup, *et al.*, 1965; Scholz and Nohl, 1976) has confirmed such diversion of fructose metabolism in the presence of ethanol.

Nevertheless, Mascord, *et al.*, (1991) observed that administration of fructose increased the rate of alcohol disposition from bloodstream by 80%, but noted an increase in lactate/pyruvate ratio. Therefore, they argued that, since fructose increased the lactate/ pyruvate ratio when it stimulates alcohol metabolism, the action of fructose cannot be explained by a decrease in the liver cytoplasmic NADH/NAD$^+$ ratio, and so, concluded that some other mechanism must be sought.

Albeit, methylene blue which attenuates the liver cytosolic increase in NADH/NAD$^+$ ratio has been reported to enhance the clearance of blood ethanol in humans (Vonlanthen, *et al.*, 2000) and this observation further strengthens the involvement of the NADH/NAD$^+$ redox and the diversion of fructose metabolism to NADH-requiring pathways in the presence of alcohol.

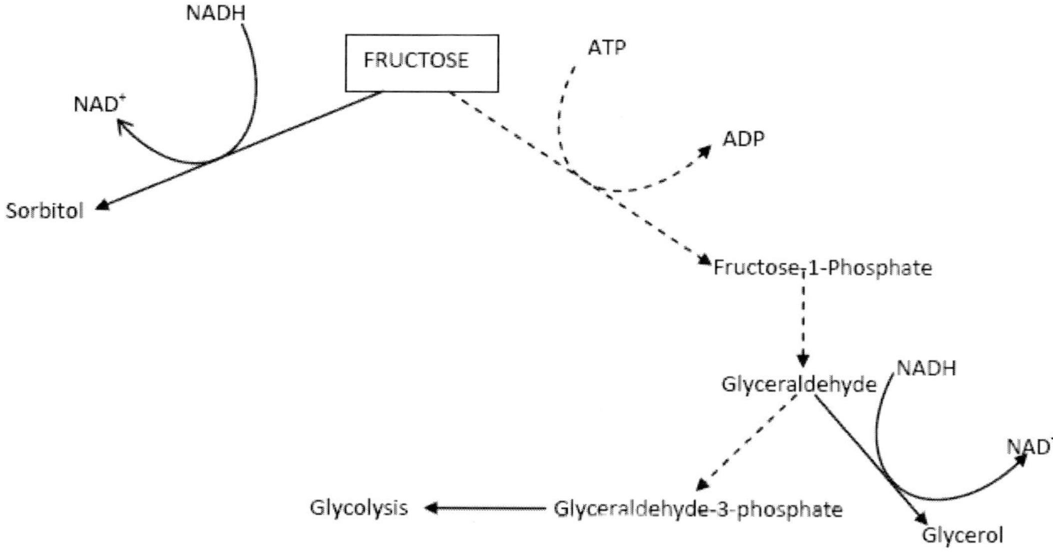

Figure 3. Hepatic metabolism of fructose in the presence (→) and absence (·········>) of ethanol (Kricka and Clark, 1979; Voet and Voet, 1995).

However, other mechanisms of the "fructose effect' have been advanced. Yamamoto *et al.* (1997) have reported that fructose enhances hepatic ATP degradation, particularly in the presence of alcohol. A fall in cellular ATP would presumably activate mitochondrial electron transport, which in turn expedites NADH oxidation to NAD$^+$. Fructose enhances hepatic ATP degradation by temporarily trapping its high energy phosphate as fructose -1- phosphate (Figure 3), and other phosphorylated glycolytic intermediates. Fructose increases the blood levels of acetaldehyde, an alcohol metabolite (Crownover, *et al.*, 1986), and the oxidation of acetaldehyde increases the mitochondrial NADH/NAD$^+$ ratio which stimulate the respiratory chain in order to re-oxidize NADH (Lieber, 1994). This may contribute to the overall "fructose effect".

Also, fructose in the stomach delays gastric emptying, and this allows increased gastric ADH oxidation (first-pass metabolism) of alcohol (Eckardt, *et al.*, 1998). This reduces the amount of alcohol absorbed and decreases its bioavailability.

Challenges of the "Fructose Effect"

The documented ability of fructose to increase the clearance of alcohol from bloodstream (fructose effect) is not without consequences. Oral administration of fructose in solution at amounts exceeding 1g/kg - the effective therapeutic dose (Berman, *et al.*, 2003) has been reported to induce gastric distress (due to malabsorption), but when given in combination with glucose, it is known to be well absorbed (Truswell, *et al.*, 1988). However, Onyesom and Ekanem (2011) have demonstrated that the co-administration of fructose and glucose to experimental animals receiving ethanol, caused increases in blood and hepatic lipids, and induced liver fibrosis.

Fructose therapy in this context, further increased blood urate (Onyesom and Anosike 2003), enhanced the levels of blood lipids and their accumulation in liver (Bantle, *et al.*, 2000; Onyesom and Anosike, 2005), affected (increased) blood pressure (Koppenol, 1998; Onyesom, 2005) and spares glucose which may cause intolerance. Research studies should be intensified in order to reduce or eliminate these and other identified side effects of the fructose therapy.

Honey and Alcohol Metabolism

Honey has been characterized to contain high amounts of fructose (30-50g) and other important nutrients like glucose (20 – 35g), thiamine, flavonoids, vitamins (Linder, *et al.*, 1996). The stimulatory effect of honey on blood alcohol oxidation has been documented (Onyesom, 2004) and were comparable with fructose, but honey's metabolic side effects were less severe (Onyesom, 2005; Onyesom, 2006). The ability of honey to ameliorate the associated metabolic disturbances may be due to its nutrients content. Flavonoids have been demonstrated to be powerful antioxidants (Siess, *et al.*, 1996), and thiamine has been reported to be involved in the metabolic detoxification of acetaldehyde (Shaw, *et al.*, 1981).

Methylene blue has been shown to prevent ethanol-induced redox changes and fat accumulation in isolated hepatocytes and HeLa cells (Galli, *et al.*, 1999) in addition to its capacity to increase the metabolism of ethanol (Vonanthen, *et al.*, 2000).

Therefore, honey or fructose fortified with antioxidants, thiamine and methylene blue may possess the potential of reducing or preventing the metabolic disturbances associated with their anti-intoxicating property and so, should be further investigated.

References

Asokan, S.K. and Witham, A.C. (1972). Myocardial malfunction of unknown cause. *Cardiovasc. Clin.* 4: 113 – 132.

Bantle, J.P., Reatz, S.K., Thomas, W. and Georgopoulos, A. (2000). Effect of dietary fructose on plasma lipids in healthy subjects. *Am. J. Clin. Nutr.* 22 : 1128 – 1134.

Berman, P.A.M., Baumgarten, I. and Vijoen, D.L. (2003). Effect of oral fructose on ethanol elimination from the bloodstream. *South Afr. J. Sci.* 99: 47 – 50.

Bora, P.S., Farrar, M.A., Miller, D.D., Chaitman, B.R. and Guruge, B.L. (1996). Myocardial cell damage by fatty acid ethyl esters. *J. Cardiovasc. Pharmacol.* 27 : 1- 6.

Brown, S.S., Forest, J.A.H. and Roscoe, P. (1972). A controlled trial of fructose in the treatment of acute alcohol intoxication. *Lancet* ii : 898 – 900.

Carpenter, T.M. and Lee, R.C. (1937). The effect of fructose on the metabolism of ethyl alcohol in man. *JPET* 60 (3): 286 – 295.

Cortot, A., Jobin, G., Ducrot, F., Aymes, C., Girandeaux, V. and Modigliani, R. (1986). Gastric emptying and gastrointestinal absorption of alcohol ingested with a meal. *Dig. Dis. Sci.* 31: 343-348.

Crownover, B.P., LaDine, J., Bradford, B., Glassman, E., Forman, D., Schneider, H. and Thurman, R.G. (1986). Activation of ethanol metabolism in humans by fructose : importance of experimental design. *J. Pharmacol. Exp. Therap.* 236 : 574 – 579.

Davies, D.L. (1973). Implications for medical practice of an acceptable concept of alcoholism. In : Alcoholism-A Medical Profile. Kessell, K., Hawkins, A., Chalke, M. and Edsall, B. (Eds.) Proceedings 1st International Federal Conference on Alcoholism, London.

Eckardt, M.J., File, S.E., Gessa, G.L., Grant, K.A., Guerri, G., Hoffinan, P.L., Kalant, H., Koob, G.F., Li, T.K. and Tabakoff, B. (1998). Effects of moderate alcohol consumption on the central nervous system. *Alcohol. Clin. Exp. Res. 22 (*25) : 998-1040.

Faller, J. and Fox, I.H. (1982). Evidence for increased urate production by activation of adenine nucleotide turnover. *N. Engl. J. Med.* 307 : 1598 – 1662.

Galli, A., Price, D. and Crabb, D. (1999). High level expression of rat class I alcohol dehydrogenase is sufficient for ethanol – induced fat accumulation in transduced HeLa cells. *Hepatology* 29 : 1164 – 1170.

Gaziano, J.M., Buring, J.E. and Breslow, J.L. (1993). Moderate alcohol intake, increased levels of high density lipoprotein and its subfractions, and decreased risk of myocardial infarction. *N. Engl. J. Med.* 329: 1829 – 1834.

Gill, J.S., Shipley, M.J., Tsementzis, S.A., Hornby, R.S., Gill, S.K. and Hitchcock, E.R. (1991). Alcohol consumption – a risk factor for hemorrhagic and non-hemorrhagic stroke. *Am. J. Med.* 90: 489-497.

Goodman, D.W. and Deykin, D. (1963). Fatty acid ethyl formation during ethanol metabolism *in vivo. Proc. Soc. Exp. Biol.* 113: 65 – 67.

Kalant, H. and Khanna, J.M. (1987). The alcohols. In : *Principles of Medical Pharmacology.* 5th (ed.), Kalant, H. and Roschlau, W.H.E. (Eds.). B.C. Decker Inc., Toronto, pp 244 – 253.

Kaplan, N.M. (1995). Alcohol and hypertension. *Lancet* 345:1588-1589.

Kei, N., Seales, J.D. and Grobbee, D.E. (1993). Alcohol intake and its relation to hypertension. *Cardiovasc. Risk Factors* 33: 189 – 200.

Knieriem, H.J. and Herbertz, G. (1969). Electron microscopic findings and photometric activation analytical results in experimental cardiac insufficiency caused by cabaltous chloride. *Virchows Arch. B. Cell. Pathol.* 2 : 32 – 46.

Koppenol, W.H. (1998). The basic chemistry of nitrogen monoxide and peroxynitrite. *Free Radic. Biol. Med.* 25 : 385 – 391.

Kricka, L.J. and Clark, P.M.S. (1979). *Biochemistry of Alcohol and Alcoholism.* Ellis Horwood Ltd., London.

Laposata, E.A and Lange, L.G. (1986). Presence of non-oxidative ethanol metabolism in human organs commonly damaged by ethanol abuse. *Science* 231:497 – 499.

Lau, P.P., Cahill, D.J., Zhu, H.J. and Chan, L. (1995). Ethanol modulates apolipoprotein B mRNA editing in the rat. *J. Lipid Res.* 86: 2069-2072.

Liang, Q., Carlson, E.C., Borgerding, A.J. and Epstein, P.N. (1999). A transgenic model of acetaldehyde overproduction accelerates alcohol cardiomyopathy. *J. Pharmacol. Exp. Therap.* 291(2): 766 – 772.

Lieber, C.S. (1991). Hepatic metabolism and toxic effects of ethanol: 1991 update. *Alcohol. Clin. Exp. Res.* 15: 573 – 592.

Lieber, C.S. (1994). Alcohol and the liver – 1994 update. *Gastroenterology* 106: 1085 – 1105.

Lieber, C.S. (1997). Ethanol metabolism, cirrhosis and alcoholism. *Clin Chim Acta* 257 (1) : 59-84.

Lieber. C.S. (1992). *Medical and Nutritional Complications of Alcoholism: Mechanisms and Management.* Plenum Press, New York.

Linder, P., Bermann, E. and Germarnik, B. (1996). Characterization of citrus honey by deuterium NMR. *J. Agric. Food Chem.* 44: 139 – 140.

Lopex, J.M., Bombi, J.A., Valderrama, R., Gimenez, A., Pares, A., Caballeria, J., Imperial, S. and Navarro, S. (1996). Effects of prolonged ethanol intake and malnutrition on rat pancreas. *Gut* 38 (2): 285 – 292.

Mascord, D., Smith, J., Starmer, G.A. and Whitfield, J.B. (1991). The effect of fructose on alcohol metabolism and the (lactate)/(pyruvate) ratio in man. *Alcohol Alcohol.* 26: 53 – 59.

Mendenhall, C.L. and Weesner, R.E. (1989). Alcoholism. In : *Clinical Chemistry.* 2nd (ed.), Kaplan, L.A. (Ed.), Amadeo J. Pesce-C.V. Mosby Company, St. Louis, pp 484 – 495.

Moushmoush, B. and Abi – Mansour, P. (1991). Alcohol and the heart : the long-term effects of alcohol on the cardiovascular system. *Arch. Intern. Med.* 151 : 36-42.

Munzinge, W. (1987). Cardiomyopathy and arsenic intoxication. *Arch. Klin. Med.* 19: 444 – 447.

National Institute on Alcohol Abuse and Alcoholism, NIAAA (1997). Alcohol metabolism. *Alcohol Alert* No. 35, Bethesda.

Neiman, J., Lang, H.E., Fornazari, L. and Carlen, P.L. (1990). Movement disorders in alcoholism: a review. *Neurology* 40 : 741 – 746.

Norton, I.D. Apte, M.V., Lux, O., Haber, P.S., Pirola, R.C. and Wilson, J.S. (1998). Chronic ethanol administration causes oxidative stress in the rat pancreas. *J. Lab. Clin. Med.* 131 (5): 442-446.

Onyesom, I. and Anosike, E.O. (2005). Effect of oral fructose on ethanol – induced changes in plasma and heptic lipids. *Acta Medica et Biologica* 53 (2): 33-36.

Onyesom, I. and Ekanem, V.J. (2011). Effect of fructose and glucose co-adminstration on ethanol – induced changes in lipids and liver morphology. *Asian J. Med. Sci.* 3 (1): 1-7.

Onyesom, I. (2003). Changes in blood pressure and plasma urate induced by the metabolism of alcohol in humans. *Global J. Med. Sci.* 2 (2): 157 – 160.

Onyesom, I. (2004). Effect of Nigerian citrus (*Citrus senensis* Osbeck) honey on ethanol metabolism. *South Afr. Med. J.* 94 (12): 984 – 986.

Onyesom, I. (2005). Honey – induced stimulation of blood ethanol elimination and its influence on serum triacylglycerol and blood pressure in man. *Ann. Nutr. Metab.* 49 :319 – 324.

Onyesom, I. (2006). Effect of natural honey on blood alcohol parameters and uric acid levels in humans. *Eur. J. Sci. Res.* 13 (3): 325- 331.

Onyesom, I. and Anosike, E.O. (2004). Oral fructose –induced disposition of blood ethanol and associated changes in plasma urate. *Afr. J. Drug Alcohol Stud* 3 (1 and 2): 21-30.

Onyesom, I. and Anosike, E.O. (2007). Changes in rabbit liver function markers after chronic exposure to ethanol. *Asian J. Biochem.* 2 (5): 337 – 342.

Onyesom, I. and Erude, H.O. (2004). Alpha amylase activity in saliva and plasma of habitual alcohol drinkers. *Biokemistri* 16 (1): 11-14.

Onyesom, I. and Naiho, A.O. (2005). Biochemical relationship between blood ethanol – generated acetaldehyde and high blood pressure in man. *West Afri. J. Biol. Sci.* 16: 22 – 28.

Onyesom, I. and Oriero, D. (2005). Effect of chronic doses of alcohol on body weight, blood glucose and lipid profile in experimental rabbits. *Alcohol Res.* 10 (6): 246 -249.

Onyesom, I., Anosike, E.O. Ebite, L.E. and Ekanem, V.J. (2007b). Changes in blood and brain glucose and lipid levels induced by ethanol and the associated microstructural alterations in brain tissue of albino rabbits. *Alcoholism* 43 (2): 71 – 79.

Onyesom, I., Onyesom, C.H., Opajobi, A.O. and Esume, C.O. (2007a). Effect of the permissive sociocultural consumption of alcohol on selected biochemical markers of liver function in serum of some Nigerian drinkers. *Adiktologie* 7 (4) : 471 – 477.

Patel, V.B., Why, H.J., Richardson, P.J. and Preedy, R. (1997). The effects of alcohol on the heart. *Adv. Drug React. Toxicol. Rev.* 16 (1) : 15 – 43.

Peters, T.J. and Preedy, V.R. (1998). Metabolic consequences of alcohol ingestion. *Novartis Found. Symp.* 216: 19- 24.

Preedy, V.R., Reilly, M.E., Patel, V.B., Richardson, P.T. and Peters, T.J. (1999). Protein metabolism in alcoholism : effects on specific tissues and the whole body. *Nutrition* 15 (7-8): 604-608.

Puddey, I.B., Rakic, V., Dimmitt, S. and Beilin, L.J. (1999). Influence of pattern of drinking on cardiovascular disease and cardiovascular risk factors. *Addiction* 94 (5): 649 – 663.

Rawat, A.K. (1974). Effectiveness of fructose in the management of alcohol withdrawal syndrome in man. In : *Alcohol and Aldehyde metabolizing Systems*. Thurman, R.G., Yonetani, T., Williamson, J.R. and Chance, B. (Eds.) Academic Press, New York, pp 313 – 323.

Rogers, J., Smith, J., Starmer, G.A. and Whitfield, J.B. (1987). Differing effects of carbohydrate, fat and protein on the rate of ethanol metabolism. *Alcohol Alcohol.* 22: 345 – 353.

Schmidt, V., Rescheleit, T., Oehmichen, M. and Schneble, H. (1995). Old wine in new bottles : the "promiller – killer " party. *Plus Blutalkohol* 32 : 241 – 253.

Scholz, R. and Nohl, H. (1976). Mechanism of the stimulatory effect of fructose on ethanol oxidation in perfused rat liver. *Eur. J. Biochem.* 63: 449- 458.

Sesso, H.D. and Gaziano, J.M. (1999). Alcohol intake and cardiovascular mortality. *Curr. Opinion Nephrol. Hypertens.* 8 (3): 353 – 357.

Shaw, S., Jayatilleke, E. and Ross, W.A. (1981). Ethanol – induced lipid peroxidation : potentiation by long-term alcohol feeding and attenuation by methionine. *J. Lab. Clin. Med.* 98:417 – 425.

Sherlock, S. (1995). Alcoholic liver disease. *Lancet* 345: 227 – 229.

Siess, M.H., Le Bon, A.M., Canivenc – Lavier, M.C., Amiot, M. J., Sabatier, S., Aubert, S.Y. and Suschetet, M. (1996). Flavonoids of honey and propolis : Characterization and effects on hepatic drug- metabolizing enzymes and benzo (a) pyrene-DNA binding in rats. *J. Agric. Food Chem.* 44:2297– 2301.

Stauhlfauth, K. and Neumaier, H. (1951). The stimulatory effect of fructose on alcohol oxidation. *Med. Klin.* 46: 590-593.

Truswell, A.S., Seach, J.M. and Thorburn, A.W. (1988). Incomplete absorption of pure fructose in healthy subjects and the facilitating effect of glucose. *Am. J. Clin. Nutr.* 48 : 1424 – 1430.

Tygstrup, N., Winkler, K. and Lunquist, F. (1965). The mechanism of the fructose effect on ethanol metabolism in human liver. *J. Clin. Invest.* 44: 817 – 830.

Urbano – Marquez, A., Estruch, R., Fernandez – Sola, J., Nicolas, J.M. Pare, J.C. and Rubin, E. (1995). The greater risk of alcoholic cardiomyopathy and myopathy in women compared with men. *J. Am. Med. Assoc.* 274 (2): 149 – 154.

Voet, D. and Voet, J.G. (1995). *Biochemistry.* 2nd (ed.), John Wiley and Sons, Inc., New York.

Vonlanthen, R., Beer, J.H. and Lauterburg, B.H. (2000). Effect of methylene blue on the disposition of ethanol. *Alcohol Alcohol.* 35 : 424 – 426.

Waldenstrom, A. (1998). Alcohol and congestive heart failure. *Alcohol. Clin. Exp. Res.* 22 (7):3153-3173.

World Health Organization, WHO (1952). *Who Tech,. Rep. Ser.*, No. 48, WHO, Geneva.

Yamamoto, T., Moriwaki, Y., Takahashi, S., Yamakita, J., Tsutsumi, Z., Ohata, H., Hiroishi, K., Nakano, T. and Higashino, K. (1997). Effect of ethanol and fructose on plasma uridine and purine bases. *Metabolism* 46 : 544 – 547.

In: Fructose
Editors: Brandon M. Johnston and Aaron B. Collins ISBN: 978-1-62081-126-9

Chapter 7

FRUCTOSE AND THE CONTROL OF FOOD INTAKE

Danielle Colley, Edra London, Baijia Jiang, Jasjeet Khural, and Thomas Castonguay*
Department of Nutrition and Food Science
University of Maryland
College Park, Maryland, US

ABSTRACT

Over the past 3 years, we have generated several lines of evidence showing that fructose can exert influence over several physiological systems that are known to participate in the regulation of food intake. In particular, we have demonstrated that fructose consumption can rapidly influence intracellular glucocorticoid regulation in both liver and adipose tissue. Further, we have reported that fructose access leads to a modification of several genes in the hypothalamus that have been linked to appetite control. The basic experimental paradigm used for these observations was to give laboratory rats free access to food, water and one of several sugar solutions for 24 h or one week, after which blood and tissues were collected. We observed that overnight fructose access (as opposed to overnight access to other sugars) leads to an almost doubling of circulating triglycerides. Despite differences in the sugars and their respective metabolic consequences, 16% (w/v) solutions of glucose, fructose and sucrose were consumed in similar amounts. All groups given access to sugar consumed significantly more calories than did rats given chow only. Diets high in fructose, but not glucose or sucrose, increased 11β-HSD1 mRNA within 24 h in both liver and adipose by greater than two- and threefold, respectively ($P \leq 0.05$). Dopamine receptors 1a and 2 and neuropeptide Y (NPY) were upregulated in the hypothalami taken from the fructose fed rats when compared to rats fed only the control diet. Hypothalamic Galanin, Brs3, AGRP, INSR, Gh1, Trhr, Atrn, NMB, TNF and Thrb were downregulated in the fructose fed group compared to controls. Results of these experiments demonstrate that fructose can have very different effects on several of the mechanisms that control food intake and body weight when compared to the effects of glucose.

---

* Correspondence: T. W. Castonguay, Ph.D. Department of Nutrition and Food Science. Rm 0112 Skinner Building. University of Maryland. College Park, MD 20742. Telephone: 301 405-4503. Email: twc@umd.edu

INTRODUCTION

Obesity has become America's most significant, preventable health problem [1, 2]. The current obesity epidemic is not attributable to any one factor, nor is it restricted by race, nationality, age or gender [3].

To date, there is no known cure for this disease. Several hypotheses about how obesity develops have been proposed. One such hypothesis is that dietary patterns of Americans have signiflcantly shifted over the past fifty years by including unprecedented amounts of refined sugar in the diet [4].

Others have added that not all sugars are the same, and that fructose in particular accounts for much of the increase in sugar intake in the American diet [5, 6]. From 1970 to 1990, consumption of high fructose corn syrup (HFCS) increased more than 1000% and currently accounts for 40% of all added caloric sweeteners [7, 8].

Evidence that fructose is capable of promoting excessive weight gain has been reported in animal models and in humans. Rats maintained on a diet rich in HFCS for 6 or 7 months show increased weight gain, increased circulating triglycerides and augmented fat deposition [9].

These observations are not without critics. Several groups have reported that when tested side-by-side, fructose is no more or less effective in promoting excess weight gain than are other sugars [10, 11].

Fructose and Obesity Animal Models

In the laboratory, sugar-induced obesity can be initiated by giving rats access to any of a wide variety of sugar solutions, where they will consume approximately 50 - 60% of their total daily caloric intake from the solution, despite differences in concentration and sweetness [12, 13, 14].

Long term access to sucrose, glucose, and fructose promotes increased weight gain and a shift in body composition favoring increased fat deposition [9]. In rats, subsequent sucrose solution restriction results in weight loss [15]. One of the most intriguing results of fructose ingestion is its effect on circulating triglycerides. Presented in Table 1 is a summary of the effects of either 1 or 7 days of access to differing 16% sugar solutions on circulating triglycerides in rats [16].

All rats had ad libitum access to diet and water. These findings replicate those previously reported in humans [17]. Recently we have repeated these measurements in another set of rats given ad lib overnight access to sucrose, fructose, glucose or High Fructose Corn Syrup (HFCS). Our observations are summarized in Figure 1.

The difference between fructose and controls was statistically significant ($P<0.05$). It is noteworthy that although the triglyceride levels in the HFCS were not statistically different from either the fructose or control groups.

Table 1. Plasma Triglycerides (mg/dl)

Dietary Group	24h access	1 wk access
Control	141.8±24.7	91.9±11.0
Sucrose	271.4± 22.6*	224.7± 31.7*
Fructose	313.5± 39.7*	276.3± 27.2*
Glucose	193.8± 21.5*	155.3± 15.7

* Significantly different from 24 h control, $P<0.05$.
(Taken from London and Castonguay [16]).

Figure 1.

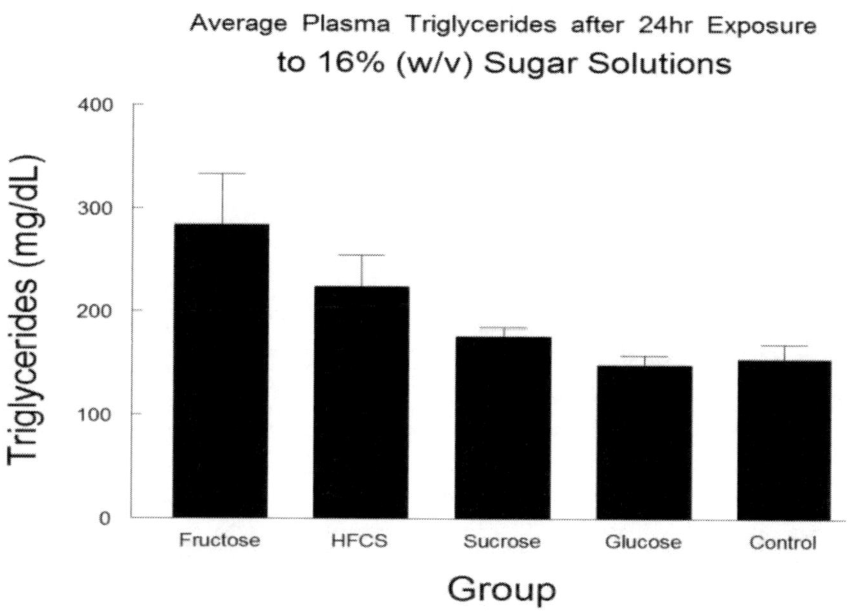

Sugar Solution Access and the Control of Food Intake

Consistent with previous observations [12], when we gave individually housed male Sprague-Dawley rats access to food water and a sugar solution they consumed a significant proportion of the day's calories as sugar. In doing so, they reduced their intake of food and increased their total daily caloric intake.

Presented in Table 2 are the mean daily intakes of diet (chow) and sugar solution. Included in the table are the calculated average solute intakes as well as the daily percentages of total intake that was consumed from sugar. Note that overnight access to fructose (F16) resulted in less sugar intake than sucrose (S16) or glucose (G16) promoted. All three groups with sugar access reduced chow intake, but the group fed fructose ate slightly more than did either of the other sugar fed groups. The net result of this adjustment was that all three groups consumed similar total calories, and all three groups ate significantly more calories than did controls.

Table 2

Group	Mean food intake (g/d)	Mean solute intake (g/d)	Mean total energy intake (kcal/d)	Mean kcal from sugar solution (%/d)
Control	25.6 ± 1.0^{A}	NA	87.3 ± 3.3^{A}	NA
S16	17.1 ± 0.9^{B}	11.7 ± 0.7^{A}	104.9 ± 4.1^{B}	44.5 ± 1.7^{A}
F16	19.7 ± 1.1^{C}	8.8 ± 0.4^{B}	102.5 ± 4.2^{B}	34.6 ± 1.7^{B}
G16	16.5 ± 0.5^{B}	11.4 ± 0.5^{A}	102.4 ± 2.1^{B}	44.9 ± 1.5^{A}

Mean daily chow, sugar solution and solute intakes; and mean daily percent of total energy from sugar solution in adult male rats given ad lib access to 16% sucrose (S16), fructose (F16) or glucose (G16) solutions in addition to chow and water for 24h. Control rats were given ad lib access to chow and water only. Different letters in columns represent differences between groups ($P < 0.05$). Taken from London and Castonguay[16].

The 11β HSD Hypothesis and Fructose

We have been interested in the role of glucocorticoids in promoting diet-induced obesity. Elevated glucocorticoids are known to promote visceral obesity and metabolic complications [18]. Circulating glucocorticoids, however, do not differ between lean and obese individuals except in cases involving Cushing's disease [19]. 11β-hydroxysteroid dehydrogenase type 1 (11β-HSD1) plays a key role in regulating tissue-specific intracellular glucocorticoids. 11β-HSD1 is a bidirectional nicotinamide adenosine dinucleotide phosphate–dependent enzyme that interconverts active and inactive glucocorticoid (20), and acts primarily as an oxo-reductase in liver and adipose thereby generating active glucocorticoid. Increased11β-HSD1 mRNA and/or activity in adipose and suppressed hepatic 11β-HSD1 mRNA and/or activity are characteristic of human and animal models of obesity. Rats fed a high-fat, high-sucrose diet in addition to an 11β-HSD1 inhibitor for 3 weeks had similar body weight and food intake as controls fed the same diet, but had reduced mesenteric adipose and adipose cell size, with no differences in epididymal or retroperitoneal fat depots [11]. An increase in 11β-HSD1 corresponds to increased reduction of 11-dehydrocorticosterone to its active form corticosterone [19, 21]. This hormone has been associated with increased gluconeogenesis and adiposity [22].

mRNA in Liver and Mesenteric Adipose 11β-HSD-1 mRNA

Recently, we have reported that in rats given overnight access to either 16% w/v sucrose, glucose or fructose solutions, only fructose increased the mean 11β-HSD1 mRNA level in liver and mesenteric adipose within the first 24h of exposure when compared to the mean levels of the control, sucrose or glucose fed controls. Continued access to fructose solution for 1 week suppressed hepatic 11β-HSD1 mRNA and increased 11β-HSD-1 mRNA in mesenteric adipose compared to controls.

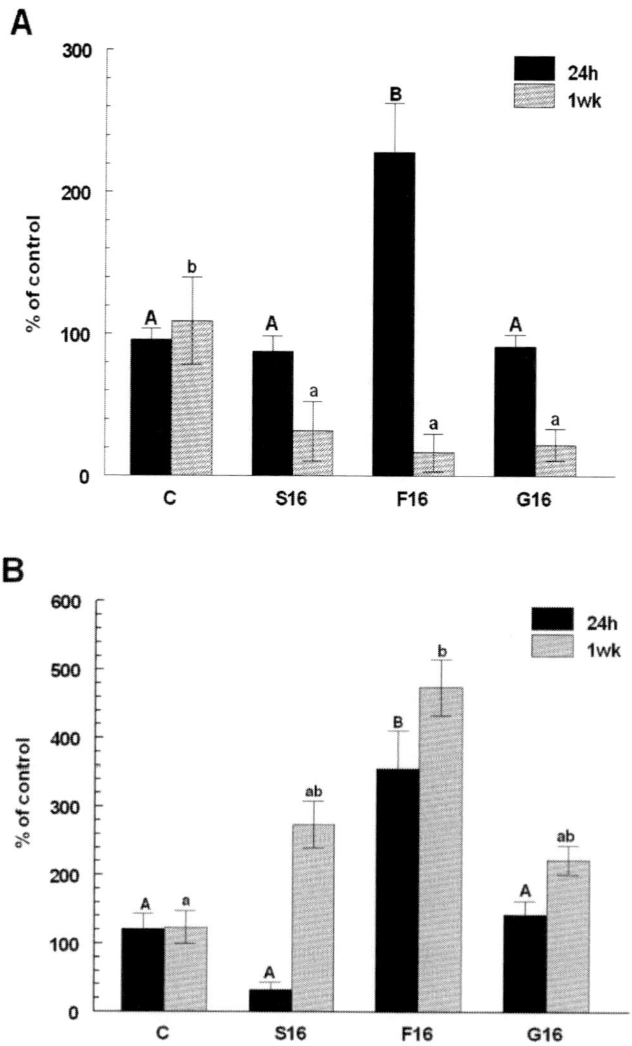

Figure 2. 11β-HSD-1 mRNA in **(A)** Liver, and **(B)** Mesenteric adipose in the control, S16, F16, and G16 groups after 24h or 1 wk exposure to the experimental diets. All data shown have been log-transformed to achieve normal distribution and graphed as the back-transformed data; values are expressed as mean ± SEM; different letters indicate a significant difference; $P< 0.05$; comparisons were made within time groups only; n= 8/gp.

After 1 wk exposure to the experimental diets, 11β-HSD-1 mRNA in liver was suppressed by greater than 60% in all the sugar-fed rats ($P< 0.05$, Fig. 2A). In mesenteric adipose the increases in 11β-HSD-1 mRNA in the sugar-fed groups at 1 wk ranged from two- to six-fold that of the control group. However, only the increased level of 11β-HSD-1 mRNA of the F16 group reached statistical significance when compared to that of the control ($P< 0.05$, Fig. 3B).

In comparing the changes in 11β-HSD-1 mRNA in response to the experimental diets, very different changes in 11β-HSD-1 mRNA were observed in the 24h and the 1 wk studies.

Figure 2A and 2B illustrate that only pure fructose solution had an immediate (24h) impact on 11β-HSD-1 mRNA in liver and mesenteric adipose. However, at 1 wk the three experimental diets had the similar effect of suppressing hepatic 11β-HSD-1 mRNA. After 1 wk, the F16 group remained the only group with significantly increased 11β-HSD-1 mRNA in adipose. An intermediate effect was seen in the other two sugar-fed groups after 1 wk as mean 11β-HSD-1 mRNA in adipose had increased relative to levels observed at 24h.

Sugar Solutions and the Hypothalamus

Despite the extensive behavioral examinations of the rat's avidity for sugar solutions, relatively little work has been focused on the impact of sugar intake on the central mechanisms controlling intake.

An exception to this characterization has been the work of Erlanson-Albertsson and colleagues, who have demonstrated that fructose can upregulate fatty acid amide hydrolase, an enzyme involved in the degredation of hypothalamic endocannabinoids, as well as other enzymes involved in the synthesis of endocannabinoids [23].

Hoebel and colleagues have reported on the pronounced effects of sugar solutions on the release of dopamine in the nucleus accumbens, the brain's so-called "reward center" [24, 25].

In addition to dopamine release, this group has demonstrated that sugar consumption can alter receptor gene expression in reward areas of the brain. Rats with intermittent sugar and chow access also have decreases in dopamine receptor D2 mRNA in the nucleus accumbens compared with *ad libitum* chow controls [26].

Bello et al have reported that sucrose intake can influence D2R density specifically in subregions of the striatum. [27]

Do Different Sugars Affect the Controls of Intake Differently?

Given the dearth of work relating sugar to changes in the CNS as well as our observations on how brief access to fructose can double circulating triglycerides and liver and adipose 11β HSD-1 expression, we next turned our attention to the neural controls of food intake, using the same experimental design where rats are given access to a dilute sugar solution overnight and compared with rats that had free access to food and water, but no sugar solution.

A number of commercially available gene-screening tools allow the investigator to monitor a large number of genes simultaneously. One such tool is a qPCR array developed by SABioscience (Gaithersburg, MD). We chose to screen the RNA extracted from the hypothalami of rats fed water, diet, and a 16% fructose solution. Controls were fed water and diet only. The rats were maintained on their respective diets overnight and then killed. At the time of sacrifice, brains were dissected and flash frozen at -80°C for subsequent analyses.

Frozen brains were sectioned using an IEC Minot Custom Microtome (Damon/IEC Division) and ten, consecutive 20 micron-thick tissue slices were sectioned from the hypothalamic region starting at the Interaural line +6.44 mm, using the Watson and Paxinos rat brain atlas as reference. Refer to Figure 3.

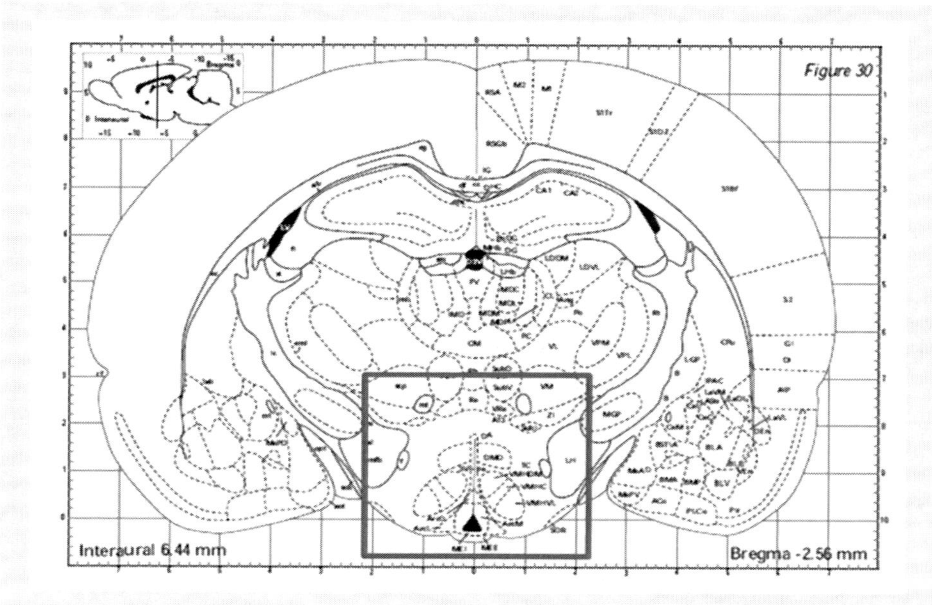

Hypothalamic areas sampled outlined in red

Table 3. Genes measured using the RT² Profiler™ PCR Obesity Array

	Orexigenic Genes	Anorectic Genes	Genes related to Energy Expenditure
Neuropeptides and Receptors	Adra2b, Agrp, Cnr1, Gal, Galr1, Mchr1 (Gpr24), Hcrt, Hcrtr1, Npy, Npy1r, Nr3c1 (Grl1), Oprk1, Oprm1, Oprs1.	Atrn (Attractin), Bdnf, Brs3, Calca, Calcr, Cart, Cntf, Cntfr, Crh, Crhr1, Drd1a, Drd2, Gh1, Ghr, Prlhr (Gpr10), Grp, Grpr, Hrh1, Htr2c, Il1a, Il1b, Il1r1, Il6, Il6ra, Mc3r, Nmb, Nmbr, Nmu, Nmur1 (Gpr66), Ntrk1, Nts, Ntsr1, Pomc, Sort1, Trh, Trhr, Ucn.	
Gut Hormone and Receptor	Ghrl (Ghrelin), Ghsr.	Apoa4, Cck, Cckar, Glp1r, Pyy.	
Adipocyte-derived Peptides and Receptors:		Lep (Leptin), Lepr, Tnf.	Adipoq (Acrp30), Adipor1, Adipor2, Adrb1, C3, Ppara, Pparg, Ppargc1a, Ptpn1, Ucp1.
Pancrease Derived Peptides and Receptors		Calcr, Clps, Gcg, Gcgr, Glp1r, Iapp, Ins1, Ins2, Insr, Ramp3, Sst, Sstr1.	
CNS-derived Peptides and Receptors			Adcyap1, Adcyap1r1, Thrb

Table 4. Effect of overnight access to fructose solution on message of appetite regulating genes. Robust changes from control (minimum 400% increase or 75% decrease)

Hypothalamic region	Gene	% of control	
		Increase	Decrease
Found in the Lateral Hypothalamus			
Glucagon-like peptide 1 receptor	Glp1R		5
Dopamine receptor D1A	Drd1a	1220	
Dopamine receptor D2	Drd2	670	
Found in the Ventromedial Hypothalamus			
Brain derived neurotrophic factor	Bdnf		2
Glucagon-like peptide 1 receptor	Glp1R		5
Dopamine receptor D1A	Drd1a	1220	
Dopamine receptor D2	Drd2	670	
Agouti related protein homolog	AGRP		0.4
Attractin	Atrn		0.4
Found in the Arcuate Nucleus			
Bombesin-like receptor 3	Brs3		5
Agouti related protein homolog	AGRP		0.4
Insulin receptor	INSR		0.9
Growth hormone 1	Gh1		2
Thyrotropin releasing hormone receptor	Trhr		3
Attractin	Atrn		0.4
Found in the Periventricular Hypothalamus			
Neuromedin B	NMB		3
Insulin receptor	INSR		0.9
Growth hormone 1	Gh1		2
Tumor necrosis factor	TNF		2
Attractin	Atrn		0.4
Thyroid hormone receptor beta	Thrb		4
Found in the Dorsomedial Hypothalamus			
Brain derived neurotrophic factor	Bdnf		2
Thyrotropin releasing hormone receptor	Trhr		3
Found in the Periventricular Thalamus			
Receptor activity modifying protein 3	Ramp3		17

We have made the somewhat arbitrary decision to include genes in this list if fructose increased message at least by 4-fold than found in control, or suppressed its expression to no more than 25% of control.

Table 5. Effect of overnight access to fructose solution. Less robust changes from control (minimum 200% increase or 50% decrease)

Hypothalamic region	Gene	% of control	
		Increase	Decrease
Found in the Lateral Hypothalamus			
Hypocretin	HCRT		36
Found in the Ventromedial Hypothalamus			
Melanin-concentrating horm receptor 1	Mchr1	270	
Found in the Arcuate Nucleus			
Neuropeptide Y	NPY	310	
Hypocretin	HCRT		36
Melanocortin 3 receptor	MC3R		37
Somatostatin receptor 1	Sstr1		4
Galanin receptor 1	GALR1		4.7
Found in the Periventricular Hypothalamus			
Thyrotropin releasing hormone	TRH		3.9
Galanin receptor 1	GALR1		4.7
Found in the Dorsomedial Hypothalamus			
Melanin-concentrating horm receptor 1	Mchr1	270	
Found in the Whole Hypothalamus			
Adenylate cyclase active.polypeptide 1	Adcyap1		4.3
Glucagon receptor	GCGR		3.8
Colipase, pancreatic	CLPS		4.3
Periventricular Thalamus			
Neuromedin B receptor	Nmbr	240	

Rat Obesity RT² Profiler™ PCR Arrays (PARN-017A) were purchased from SABiosciences (Frederick, MD). Each array profiled the expression of 84 genes related to obesity, including genes that code for orexigenic peptides, hormones, and receptors, anorectic peptides, hormones, and receptors, and central and peripheral signaling molecules related to energy expenditure. See Table 2 for the complete list of genes included in the arrays.

Hypothalamic cDNA templates were pooled by diet so that differences attributable to only the difference in diet could clearly be measured. Diluted First Strand cDNA was added to the 2X SABiosciences RT^2 qPCR Master Mix and aliquoted into each of 96-wells of the obesity arrays. Arrays were run according to the SABiosciences protocol: 95°C for 10 min, and 40 cycles at 95°C, 15 s; and 60°C, 1 min. Results were analyzed using the SABioscience's online RT² Profiler™ PCR Array.

Dopamine receptors 1a and 2 and neuropeptide Y (NPY) were upregulated in the hypothalami taken from the fructose fed group compared to control. Galanin, Brs3, AGRP, INSR, Gh1, Trhr, Atrn, NMB, TNF and Thrb were downregulated in the fructose fed group.

Presented in Table 4 are the results of comparisons between fructose fed and control fed groups that were particularly pronounced.

In the table each gene is linked with a region of the hypothalamus, based upon localization (typically in situ hybridization) studies supplied by Pub Med for each gene. A second list of differences that were attributable to fructose consumption is presented in Table

5. Genes in this "less robust" list were included if message was at least doubled, or was suppressed by 50%. Note that several well-established appetite regulating genes are included in this second "less robust" list, including Hypocretin, Neuropeptide Y and Neuromedin B receptor.

CONCLUSION

The experiments presented in this review reveal that fructose can have very pronounced and distinctive effects (compared to other sugars) on several of the mechanisms that control food intake, body weight and body composition. We have demonstrated that not only does fructose uniquely promote increased circulating triglycerides, but that it can do so quickly (overnight). These changes in circulating lipid may or may not be related to the acute changes in 11β HSD1 observed in the liver and in adipose tissue, but it is notable that both changes are unique to fructose consumption, and both can be observed in a short time and with limited intake. Rats eating the same amount of other sugars (glucose or sucrose) were not comparably affected. Preliminary direct comparisons of sucrose to HFCS that are on-going in our laboratory have failed to reveal any significant differences from sucrose and glucose in many of these end points.

There are several additional findings presented here that need one final mention. First, despite differences in taste and in pathways involved in metabolizing different sugars, all of the groups consumed comparable amounts of sugar and at the same time reduced chow intake comparably. Although these adjustments have been observed with glucose, sucrose and starch [13], the data presented here extend the observations to include fructose. We have previously noted that despite differences in concentration, sucrose solutions are consumed so as to result in the same number of grams of solute consumed in any one day [13]. In previous work, we noted that additional finer adjustments in caloric intake take place over the course of then next 5-10 days, so that the proportions of sugar and diet remain the same, but total caloric intake (that typically increased 10-15% with initial sugar access) is restored to control levels (ad lib chow but without sugar solution access). The work reported in this paper is limited mostly to the first 24h of access to different solutions, a period when total caloric intake was increasing, and chow intake decreasing. We believe that it is reasonable to expect that different hypothalamic mechanisms could be involved in these separate adjustments. These will be discussed below.

Before doing so, however, it needs to be pointed out that fructose access not only affects intake, but it also promotes changes in both hepatic and adipose metabolism that are conducive to increased fat deposition. London and Castonguay [16] reported that fructose was the only sugar tested to increase hepatic and adipose 11β HSD1 message within 24h of access. Seckl [22] and Livingstone [19] have reported that obese people have decreased hepatic 11β HSD1 and increased adipose tissue 11β HSD1 message, a pattern that was observed with all 3 sugars tested after 7 days of access [16]. It remains uncertain if the additional period of elevated 11β HSD1 message promoted by fructose contributes to subsequent changes in body composition or weight gain. It has already been reported that long-term fructose access can promote increased fat deposition, compared to a control group fed only a standard diet [9].

Finally, the PCR Array analyses revealed a number of genes that were either dramatically up regulated or silenced by overnight access to fructose. We are currently conducting a more complete examination and comparison of fructose with HFCS, sucrose and glucose, to better determine which of the many fructose effects reported here are unique to fructose. The data reported here include the observation that fructose can up regulate genes in the hypothalamus associated with the dopaminergic pathways. Hoebel and his group [24] postulated that these neurons are part of the dopamine pathway involved with reward. Using different methodologies, Smith and his group reported similar conclusions – hypothalamic dopamine plays an integral role in the control of sucrose intake [28-30]. In the preliminary array scan reported here, overnight access to fructose led to significant up regulation in the message for both Dopamine 1 and 2 receptors, consistent with their conclusions using microdialysis or dopamine antagonists.

The significance of this observation is that both fructose and sucrose have an effect on this dopaminergic system, despite their separate metabolic fates. It is tempting to conclude that sensory properties associated with the intake of both sugars are determining this component of the response to the sugars. By contrast, the suppression of genes in the hypothalamus that are related to insulin (GLP1r, INSR, AGRP, and MCRh1 to name but a few), suggests that other processes are involved. Presumably some of these endpoints are also part of the regulatory system involved in promoting increased intake, while others may be more involved in adjusting chow intake subsequent to the influx of calories from fructose. Only a more in depth side-by-side comparison of the effects of different sugars will permit attribution to which of the changes reported here are specific to fructose, and which are common to sugars. Additional experiments are being planned that will better determine which of these effects are due to increased caloric intake, and which are attributable to reduced chow intake.

Acknowledgment

This work was supported in part by a competitive grant from the Maryland Agricultural Experiment Station to TWC as well as a Wylie Dissertation fellowship awarded to EL. B. Jiang and J. Khural were supported in part by the Howard Hughes Medical Foundation. Requests for reprints should be addressed to TWC.

References

[1] Jia H, Lubetkin EI. Trends in quality-adjusted life-years lost contributed by smoking and obesity. *Am. J. Prev. Med.*, 2010;38(2):138-44.

[2] Flegal KM, Carroll MD, Ogden CL, Curtin LR. Prevalence and trends in obesity among US adults, 1999-2008. *JAMA*. 2010;303(3):235-41.

[3] Canoy D, Buchan I. Challenges in obesity epidemiology. *Obes. Rev.*, 2007;8 Suppl 1:1-11.

[4] Paeratakul S, York-Crowe EE, Williamson DA, Ryan DH, Bray GA. Americans on diet: results from the 1994-1996 Continuing Survey of Food Intakes by Individuals. *J. Am. Diet. Assoc.*, 2002;102(9):1247-51.

[5] Johnson RJ, Segal MS, Sautin Y, Nakagawa T, Feig DI, Kang DH, et al. Potential role of sugar (fructose) in the epidemic of hypertension, obesity and the metabolic syndrome, diabetes, kidney disease, and cardiovascular disease. *Am. J. Clin. Nutr.*, 2007;86(4):899-906.

[6] van Dam RM, Seidell JC. Carbohydrate intake and obesity. *Eur. J. Clin. Nutr.*, 2007;61 Suppl 1:S75-99.

[7] Bray GA, Paeratakul S, Popkin BM. Dietary fat and obesity: a review of animal, clinical and epidemiological studies. *Physiol. Behav.*, 2004;83(4):549-55.

[8] Bray GA. Fructose: pure, white, and deadly? Fructose, by any other name, is a health hazard. *J. Diabetes. Sci. Technol.*, 2010;4(4):1003-7.

[9] Bocarsly ME, Powell ES, Avena NM, Hoebel BG. High-fructose corn syrup causes characteristics of obesity in rats: increased body weight, body fat and triglyceride levels. *Pharmacol. Biochem. Behav.*, 2010;97(1):101-6.

[10] Melanson KJ, Angelopoulos TJ, Nguyen V, Zukley L, Lowndes J, Rippe JM. High-fructose corn syrup, energy intake, and appetite regulation. *Am. J. Clin. Nutr.*, 2008;88(6):1738S-44S.

[11] Soenen S, Westerterp-Plantenga MS. No differences in satiety or energy intake after high-fructose corn syrup, sucrose, or milk preloads. *Am. J. Clin. Nutr.*, 2007;86(6):1586-94.

[12] Collier G, Bolles R. Some determinants of intake of sucrose solutions. *J. Comp. Physiol. Psychol.*, 1968;65(3):379-83.

[13] Castonguay TW, Hirsch E, Collier G. Palatability of sugar solutions and dietary selection? *Physiol. Behav.*, 1981;27(1):7-12.

[14] Hill W, Castonguay TW, Collier GH. Taste or diet balancing? *Physiol. Behav.*, 1980;24(4):765-7.

[15] Hirsch E, Walsh M. Effect of limited access to sucrose on overeating and patterns of feeding. *Physiol. Behav.*, 1982;29(1):129-34.

[16] London E, Castonguay TW. High fructose diets increase 11β-hydroxysteroid dehydrogenase type 1 in liver and visceral adipose in rats within 24-h exposure. *Obesity*, (*Silver Spring*). 2011;19(5):925-32.

[17] Teff KL, Elliott SS, Tschöp M, Kieffer TJ, Rader D, Heiman M, et al. Dietary fructose reduces circulating insulin and leptin, attenuates postprandial suppression of ghrelin, and increases triglycerides in women. *J. Clin. Endocrinol. Metab.*, 2004;89(6):2963-72.

[18] Tomlinson JW, Walker EA, Bujalska IJ, Draper N, Lavery GG, Cooper MS, et al. 11beta-hydroxysteroid dehydrogenase type 1: a tissue-specific regulator of glucocorticoid response. *Endocr. Rev.*, 2004;25(5):831-66.

[19] Livingstone DE, Jones GC, Smith K, Jamieson PM, Andrew R, Kenyon CJ, et al. Understanding the role of glucocorticoids in obesity: tissue-specific alterations of corticosterone metabolism in obese Zucker rats. *Endocrinology*, 2000;141(2):560-3.

[20] Seckl JR. 11beta-Hydroxysteroid dehydrogenase in the brain: a novel regulator of glucocorticoid action? Front *Neuroendocrinol.*, 1997;18(1):49-99.

[21] Czegle I, Margittai E, Senesi S, Benedetti A, Bánhegyi G. Different expression and distribution of 11beta-hydroxysteroid dehydrogenase type 1 in obese and lean animal models of type 2 diabetes. *Acta. Physiol. Hung.*, 2008;95(4):419-24.

[22] Seckl JR. Glucocorticoids, developmental 'programming' and the risk of affective dysfunction. *Prog. Brain Res.*, 2008;167:17-34.

[23] Erlanson-Albertsson C, Lindqvist A. Fructose affects enzymes involved in the synthesis and degradation of hypothalamic endocannabinoids. *Regul. Pept.*, 2010;161(1-3):87-91.

[24] Avena NM, Bocarsly ME, Rada P, Kim A, Hoebel BG. After daily bingeing on a sucrose solution, food deprivation induces anxiety and accumbens dopamine/ acetylcholine imbalance. *Physiol. Behav.*, 2008;94(3):309-15.

[25] Rada P, Avena NM, Hoebel BG. Daily bingeing on sugar repeatedly releases dopamine in the accumbens shell. *Neuroscience*, 2005;134(3):737-44.

[26] Spangler R, Wittkowski KM, Goddard NL, Avena NM, Hoebel BG, Leibowitz SF. Opiate-like effects of sugar on gene expression in reward areas of the rat brain. *Brain Res. Mol. Brain Res.*, 2004;124(2):134-42.

[27] Bello NT, Lucas LR, Hajnal A. Repeated sucrose access influences dopamine D2 receptor density in the striatum. *Neuroreport*, 2002;13(12):1575-8.

[28] Simansky KJ, Bourbonais KA, Smith GP. Food-related stimuli increase the ratio of 3,4-dihydroxyphenylacetic acid to dopamine in the hypothalamus. *Pharmacol. Biochem. Behav.*, 1985;23(2):253-8.

[29] Smith GP, Bourbonais KA, Jerome C, Simansky KJ. Sham feeding of sucrose increases the ratio of 3,4-dihydroxyphenylacetic acid to dopamine in the hypothalamus. *Pharmacol. Biochem. Behav.*, 1987;26(3):585-91.

[30] Weatherford SC, Greenberg D, Gibbs J, Smith GP. The potency of D-1 and D-2 receptor antagonists is inversely related to the reward value of sham-fed corn oil and sucrose in rats. *Pharmacol. Biochem. Behav.*, 1990;37(2):317-23.

ABBREVIATIONS

Brs3- bombesin-like receptor 3,
AGRP- agouti related protein homolog,
INSR- insulin receptor,
Gh1- growth hormone 1,
Trhr- thyrotropin releasing hormone receptor,
Atrn- attractin,
NMB- neuromedin B,
TNF- tumor necrosis factor,
Thrb- thyroid hormone receptor beta,
CCK- cholecystokinin,
Ucn- urocortin,
ADR2B- adrenergic, alpha-2B-, receptor,
NTKR1- neurotrophic tyrosine kinase, receptor, type 1,
ADIPOQ- adiponectin,
IAPP- islet amyloid polypeptide

In: Fructose
Editors: Brandon M. Johnston and Aaron B. Collins
ISBN: 978-1-62081-126-9

Chapter 8

EFFECT OF FRUCTOSE ON HEALTH

Tzi Bun Ng[1], Jack Ho Wong[1], Evandro Fei Fang[1], and Xiujuan Ye[2]
[1]School of Biomedical Sciences, Faculty of Medicine, The Chinese University of Hong Kong, Hong Kong,China
[2]Institute of Plant Virology, Fujian Province Key Laboratory of Plant Virology, Fujian Agriculture and Forestry University, Fuzhou, Fujian, China

ABSTRACT

Fructose and fructose-based sweeteners are the most commonly added sugars in our diet. Fructose has both beneficial actions as well as harmful effects.Lactulose formed by lactose isomerization, stimulates the growth of health-promoting bacteria in the gastrointestinal tract, and suppresses proliferation of pathogenic bacteria. Calcium fructoborate reduces exacerbated cellular immune responses induced by mycotoxins from *Fusarium* species. Fructooligosaccharides have probiotic effect, improve mineral absorption, reduce constipation, and reduce serum levels of cholesterol, triacylglycerols and phospholipids. They are additives in some food products and infant formulas due to their probiotic effect. Fructose is a highly lipogenic nutrient implicated in insulin resistance, hepatic steatosis, and the metabolic syndrome. Fructose induces an increase in ethanol metabolism and elevates the risk of Syndrome X. A high-fructose diet aggravates eccentric left ventricular hypertrophy in experimental volume overload.The diet also results in development of hypertension. Excessive dietary carbohydrates, especially fructose, may promote the development of Alzheimer's disease. An excess of carbohydrates, such as fructose and chocolate, either during gestation or lactation, has an adverse effect on offspring.Maternal fructose intake during pregnancy and lactation alters placental growth and leads to sex-specific changes in fetal and neonatal endocrine function. The aqueous extract of *Globularia alypum* decreases hypertriglyceridemia and ameliorates oxidative status of the muscle, kidney, and heart in rats fed a high-fructose diet. Grape seed extract supplementation prevents high-fructose diet-induced insulin resistance in rats by improving insulin and adiponectin signalling pathways. Despite the evidence presented above, some investigators are of the opinion that there is insufficient evidence to support the prohibition or restriction of the use of high fructose corn syrup or other fructose-containing sweeteners or to advocate the use of warning labels on products containing high fructose corn syrup.

Although some studies indicate that fructose does not bring about biologically relevant changes in triglyceride or body weight when consumed at levels near 95th percentile estimates of intake, it is advisable to restrict ingestion of caloric sweeteners, including high fructose corn syrup.

INTRODUCTION

Fructose has become a major constituent of the human diet. The main sources are sucrose from cane and beet , high fructose corn syrup, honey and fruits.Although fructose and glucose share the same chemical formula, fructose metabolism is distinct from glucose metabolism owing to the nearly complete hepatic extraction of fructose and its speedy hepatic transformation into glucose, glycogen, lactate, and fat. Initially fructose was deemed to be recommendable to diabetic patients because of its low glycemic index. However, consumption of large amounts of fructose in rodents over a long period elicits high blood pressure, obesity, hepatic and extrahepatic insulin resistance, and type 2 diabetes mellitus.In humans, high fructose intake causes dyslipidemia and attenuates hepatic insulin sensitivity. However, unequivocal evidence that moderate fructose intake exerts adverse metabolic effects is lacking. There is no direct evidence that consumption of high fructose corn syrup produces more serious metabolic consequences than intake of sucrose (Tappy and Lê,2010).In the following, the beneficial as well as deleterious effects of fructose are discussed.

BENEFICIAL EFFECTS OF FRUCTOSE

Lactulose Stimulates the Growth of Health-Promoting Bacteria in the Gastrointestinal Tract, and Inhibits Growth of Pathogenic Bacteria

Lactulose, a "bifidus factor", formed by lactose isomerization, comprises galactose and fructose. It is a prebiotic carbohydrate that exerts growth-promoting effects on beneficial bacteria in the gastrointestinal tract, such as bifidobacteria and lactobacilli and growth-suppressing effects on pathogenic bacteria such as Salmonella. It can also be employed for the treatment of constipation and hepatic encephalopathy, tumour prevention, and for maintenance of blood glucose and insulin levels. It has potential applications in food and pharmaceutical industries (Panesar and Kumari, 2011).

Dietary Fructooligosaccharides and Potential Benefits on Health

Fructooligosaccharides (FOS) are naturally occuring oligosaccharides found in artichoke, asparagus, banana, chicory, garlic, onion, and many other plants. They are composed of linear chains of 2 to 60 fructose units, connected by beta (2-1) bonds. Dietary FOS are not hydrolyzed by glycosidases in the small intestine and go to the cecum structurally unaltered.

They are metabolized by intestinal microflora to yield CO(2), hydrogen, L-lactate, short-chain carboxylic acids, and other metabolites. FOS have a low sweetness; are calorie-free, non-cariogenic and are considered as soluble dietary fibre. Furthermore, FOS have low carcinogenicity and probiotic effect, improve mineral absorption and reduce serum levels of cholesterol, triacylglycerols and phospholipids. FOS are added to some food products and infant formulas due to their probiotic effect. Their consumption reduce constipation (Sabater-Molina et al.,2009).

Calcium Fructoborate Reduces Exacerbated Cellular Immune Responses Induced by Fusarium Toxins

Trichotecenes are toxins produced by *Fusarium* sp., found as contaminants in human food and animal feeds. Taranu et al.(2011) performed a feeding trial to assess the effect of a fusarotoxin-contaminated diet, and to investigate the counteracting action of a calcium fructoborate additive on performance and immune response in weaned pigs. Maize contaminated with low doses of *Fusarium* mycotoxins including deoxynivalenol, T-2/HT-2 toxins, zearalenone, and fumonisins (1790, 90, 20, and 0·6 parts per billion) was included in a maize-soyabean meal diet, and provided *ad libitum* to weaned piglets for 24 d. Supplementation with calcium fructoborate ameliorated the decrease in performance seen in contaminated animals, and reduced the exacerbated cellular immune responses induced by *Fusarium* toxins including increased ex vivo peripheral blood mononuclear cell proliferation, respiratory burst of porcine granulocytes, percentage of peripheral T, CD3(+), CD3(+)CD4(+) andCD3(+)CD8(+) subsets and the synthesis of TNF-α, IL-1β, and IL-8.

DELETERIOUS EFFECTS OF FRUCTOSE

The Role of Fructose-Enriched Diets in Mechanisms of Nonalcoholic Fatty Liver Disease

Fructose, a major dietary caloric sweetener, is implicated in the pathogenesis of nonalcoholic fatty liver disease (NAFLD),a benign form of liver dysfunction. Inflammatory progression to nonalcoholic steatohepatitis (NASH) which may lead to liver cirrhosis and hepatocellular carcinoma, takes place by a two-hit process. The first "hit" involves accumulation of fat in the liver caused by enhanced de novo lipogenesis, suppression of fatty acid beta-oxidation, impaired triglyceride clearance and reduced export of very-low-density lipoprotein.

The possible mechanisms of the second "hit" comprise inflammation brought about by oxidative stress associated with lipid peroxidation, cytokine activation, nitric oxide and reactive oxygen species, and endogenous toxins of fructose metabolites(Nomura and Yamanouchi,2011).

Fructose: A Highly Lipogenic Nutrient Implicated in Insulin Resistance, Hepatic Steatosis, and the Metabolic Syndrome

Fructose is a highly lipogenic sugar with metabolic effects and associated with components of the metabolic syndrome (insulin resistance, elevated waist circumference, dyslipidemia, and hypertension). Fructose feeding changes gene expression patterns (such as hepatic peroxisome proliferator-activated receptor-γ coactivator-1α/β) and satiety factors in the brain. It increases inflammation, reactive oxygen species, and portal endotoxin concentrations via Toll-like receptors, and brings about leptin resistance. It leads to the development of insulin resistance, hepatic steatosis, and the metabolic syndrome(Dekker et al.,2011).

Fructose-Induced Increase in Ethanol Metabolism and the Risk of Syndrome X

Fructose and alcohol increase the risk of Syndrome X characterized by high blood pressure, altered HDL-cholesterol content, hypertriglyceridemia, and impaired glucose tolerance. Administration of fructose (1 g fructose/kg body weight) shortened the duration of alcohol intoxication in light alcohol drinkers (<20 g/day) between the ages of 25 and 35 years by 30.7%, and speeded up alcohol elimination (metabolism) from blood by 44.7%. However,ethanol together with fructose increased the number of subjects with impaired glucose and triglyceride levels to 13 (29%) and 43 (96%) from 8 (18%) and 37 (82%) caused by ethanol alone. If the anti-ethanol intoxicating activity of fructose to be exploited, the problem of metabolic syndrome associated with oral fructose has to be dealt with (Uzuegbu and Onyesom,2009).

Metabolic and Behavioural Effects of Sucrose and Fructose/Glucose Drinks

Rats with access to sugar-sweetened beverages displayed larger abdominal fat pads, higher triglyceride levels and exhibited impaired insulin/glucose homeostasis. Fasting hyperglycaemia was found in the fructose-glucose treated group, but not in sucrose-treated group.The sucrose-treated group exhibited increased activity in an open field. Thus 'free' fructose poses a greater risk of progression to type 2 diabetes than 'bound' fructose (sucrose) (Sheludiakova et al.,2011).

Fructose elevates lipogenesis, triglycerides, and blood pressure, but exhibits a smaller effect on leptin and insulin release compared to glucose. In controlled feeding studies, fat storage, triglycerides and body weight were altered together with an increase in inflammatory markers. It is believed that fructose is hazardous to the cardiometabolic health (Bray,2010).

However,Sun et al.(2011) reported that fructose intake and intake of non-fructose sugar were not positively correlated with the waist circumference, body mass index, blood pressure, and blood concentrations of glycated hemoglobin, HDL-cholesterol, triglyceride, and uric acid, in the adults studied (aged 19 to 80, n=17,749).

Fructose and Changes in Triglyceride or Body Weight

Triglyceride concentrations are elevated and concentrations of insulin and satiety-associated hormones are reduced in experimental animals after consumption of fructose.By contrast, data from human studies are inconsistent probably due to dependence on the particular study population, the design of the studies, and/or the amount of fructose ingested. The results indicate that fructose does not bring about biologically relevant changes in triglyceride or body weight when consumed at levels near 95th percentile estimates of intake(Dolan et al.,2010).

A High-Fructose Diet Worsens Eccentric Left Ventricular Hypertrophy in Experimental Volume Overload

A fructose-rich diet produced in rats a deterioration of left ventricular eccentric hypertrophy and reduced left ventricular function in a model of chronic volume overload brought about by aortic valve regurgitation. Normal rats fed the same diet did not exhibit these abnormalities.

Hypertriglyceridemia may play a central role in this phenomenon (Bouchard-Thomassin et al.,2011).

Fructose and Hypertension

Overactivation of the sympathetic nervous system, augmented generation of vasoconstrictors including endothelin-1, angiotensin II, and prostanoids, and impaired endothelium-dependent relaxation, increased formation of reactive oxygen species and elevated levels of uric acid play a role in the development of hypertension in fructose-fed rats. (Tran et al.,2009).

Nutrition and Alzheimer's Disease: The Detrimental Role of a High Carbohydrate Diet

Excessive dietary carbohydrates, especially fructose, coupled with a relative deficiency in dietary fats and cholesterol, may lead to the development of Alzheimer's disease. The initial step in the pathophysiology of Alzheimer's disease is formation of advanced glycation end-products in plasma proteins involved in transport of fat, cholesterol, and oxygen. The resulting cholesterol deficiency impairs neuronal function. A cascade response ensues in impaired glutamate signaling, increased oxidative damage, lysosomal and mitochondrial dysfunction, elevated risk to microbial infection, and, eventually, apoptosis. (Seneff et al.,2011).

Increased Fructose Intake as a Risk Factor for Dementia

T A diet transition in the United States has occurred in the intake of refined sugar, particularly high-fructose corn syrup from a yearly estimate of 8.1 kg/person at the beginning of the XIX century to a current estimate of 65 kg/person. This article considers the association between refined sugar intake, markers of cardiovascular disease risk, and the possible promotion of the development of dementia (Stephan et al.,2010).

Aqueous Extract of Globularia Alypum Decreases Hypertriglyceridemia and Ameliorates Oxidative Status of the Muscle, Kidney, and Heart in Rats Fed a High-Fructose Diet

A high-fructose diet in rats elevated plasma levels of triglycerides and very low-density lipoprotein-triglyceride, and thiobarbituric acid-reactive substances in the liver, muscle, and heart. On the other hand, hepatic and cardiac superoxide dismutase, hepatic catalase and cardiac glutathione peroxidase activities declined. The aqueous extract of Globularia alypum lowered the levels of triglycerides in very low-density lipoprotein and high-density lipoprotein . Levels of renal and muscle thiobarbituric acid-reactive substance were reduced. Superoxide dismutase activity in the muscle and heart, and glutathione peroxidase activity in the kidney and heart was increased (Taleb-Dida et al.,2011).

Grape Seed Extract Supplementation Prevents High-Fructose Diet-Induced Insulin Resistance in Rats By Improving Insulin and Adiponectin Signalling Pathways

In rats a high-fructose diet brought about insulin resistance by downregulating the protein expression of insulin receptor, insulin receptor substrate-1, Akt and GLUT4, and the mRNA expression of adiponectin, adiponectin receptor R1 and AMP-activated protein kinase (AMPK)-α in the skeletal muscle. Supplementation with grape seed extract had an ameliorating action.It enhanced the expression of insulin signalling pathway-related proteins, including Akt and GLUT4, augmented the mRNA expression of adiponectin, adiponectin receptor R1, AMPK-α, and glycogen synthase, and downregulated the mRNA expression of glycogen synthase kinase-3-α, leading to glycogen accumulation in the skeletal muscle. (Meeprom et al.,2011).

Effects of a Maternal Diet Supplemented with Chocolate and Fructose Beverage during Gestation and Lactation on Rat Dams and their Offspring

An excess of carbohydrates, such as fructose and chocolate, either during gestation or lactation, has an adverse effect on the offspring (Zhang et al.,2011).

Maternal Fructose Intake during Pregnancy and Lactation Alters Placental Growth and Leads to Sex-Specific Changes in Fetal and Neonatal Endocrine Function

In rats, maternal consumption led to sex-specific changes in offspring development. Female offsprings were more susceptible to metabolic compromise than males during the neonatal period. Placental weights were reduced in female but not male fetuses. Plasma fructose, glucose and leptin levels were elevated and β-hydroxybutyrat reduced in female but not male fetuses (Vickers et al.,2011).

DISCUSSION

In the small intestine, the disaccharide sucrose is easily broken down, and thus free fructose and glucose are absorbed from both sucrose and high fructose corn syrup. To the food manufacturers, compared to sucrose, the free monosaccharides in high fructose corn syrup provide better flavor enhancement, color, freshness, stability, texture, pourability, and consistency in foods.Fructose and fructose-based sweeteners are the most commonly added sugars. High-fructose corn syrup is a major added caloric sweetener. However, in comparison with other caloric sweeteners, consumption of high fructose corn syrup may elevate the risk for obesity and other adverse health consequences. Knowledge of the effect of fructose overconsumption in the development of metabolic disorders may be used in the developing of strategies aimed at preventing unhealthy dietary behavior and thus the increasing trend in insulin resistance, obesity and diabetes (Collino,2011).On the other hand, Moeller et al.(2009) were of the opinion that since high fructose corn syrup and sucrose are similar in composition, especially upon absorption by the body, it is not very likely that high fructose corn syrup induces obesity or other conditions more than sucrose. There is insufficient evidence to support prohibiting or restricting the use of high fructose corn syrup or other fructose-containing sweeteners or to advocate the use of warning labels on products containing high fructose corn syrup. Nevertheless, it is advisable to restrict ingestion of caloric sweeteners, including high fructose corn syrup .

REFERENCES

Bouchard-Thomassin AA, Lachance D, Drolet MC, Couet J, Arsenault M. A high-fructose diet worsens eccentric left ventricular hypertrophy in experimental volume overload. *Am. J. Physiol. Heart Circ. Physiol.* 2011 ;300(1):H125-34.

Bray GA. Soft drink consumption and obesity: it is all about fructose. *Curr. Opin. Lipidol.* 2010 ;21(1):51-.

Collino M. High dietary fructose intake: Sweet or bitter life? *World J. Diabetes.* 2011;2(6):77-81.

Dekker MJ, Su Q, Baker C, Rutledge AC, Adeli K. Fructose: a highly lipogenic nutrient implicated in insulin resistance, hepatic steatosis, and the metabolic syndrome. *Am. J. Physiol. Endocrinol. Metab.* 2010 ;299(5):E685-94.

Dolan LC, Potter SM, Burdock GA. Evidence-based review on the effect of normal dietary consumption of fructose on development of hyperlipidemia and obesity in healthy, normal weight individuals. *Crit. Rev. Food. Sci. Nutr.* 2010 ;50(1):53-84.

Meeprom A, Sompong W, Suwannaphet W, Yibchok-anun S, Adisakwattana S. Grape seed extract supplementation prevents high-fructose diet-induced insulin resistance in rats by improving insulin and adiponectin signalling pathways. *Br. J. Nutr.* 2011;106(8):1173-81.

Moeller SM, Fryhofer SA, Osbahr AJ 3rd, Robinowitz CB The effects of high fructose syrup. *J. Am. Coll. Nutr.* 2009 ;28(6):619-26.

Nomura K, Yamanouchi T. The role of fructose-enriched diets in mechanisms of nonalcoholic fatty liver disease. *J. Nutr. Biochem.* 2011 Nov 28.

Panesar PS, Kumari S. Lactulose: production, purification and potential applications. *Biotechnol. Adv.* 2011;29(6):940-8.

Sabater-Molina M, Larqué E, Torrella F, Zamora S. Dietary fructooligosaccharides and potential benefits on health. *J. Physiol. Biochem.* 2009 ;65(3):315-28.

Seneff S, Wainwright G, Mascitelli L. Nutrition and Alzheimer's disease: the detrimental role of a high carbohydrate diet. *Eur. J. Intern. Med.* 2011 ;22(2):134-40.

Sheludiakova A, Rooney K, Boakes RA. Metabolic and behavioural effects of sucrose and fructose/glucose drinks in the rat. *Eur. J. Nutr.* 2011 Jul 29. [Epub ahead of print].

Stephan BC, Wells JC, Brayne C, Albanese E, Siervo M.Increased fructose intake as a risk factor for dementia. *J. Gerontol A Biol. Sci. Med. Sci.* 2010 ;65(8):809-14.

Sun SZ, Anderson GH, Flickinger BD, Williamson-Hughes PS, Empie MW. Fructose and non-fructose Taleb-Dida N, Krouf D, Bouchenak M. Globularia alypum aqueous extract decreases hypertriglyceridemia and ameliorates oxidative status of the muscle, kidney, and heart in rats fed a high-fructose diet. *Nutr. Res.* 2011 ;31(6):488-95.

Tappy L, Lê KA. Metabolic effects of fructose and the worldwide increase in obesity. *Physiol. Rev.* 2010;90(1):23-46.

Taranu I, Marin DE, Manda G, Motiu M, Neagoe I, Tabuc C, Stancu M, Olteanu M. Assessment of the potential of a boron-fructose additive in counteracting the toxic effect of Fusarium mycotoxins. *Br. J. Nutr.* 2011 ;106(3):398-407.

Tran LT, Yuen VG, McNeill JH. The fructose-fed rat: a review on the mechanisms of fructose-induced insulin resistance and hypertension. *Mol Cell Biochem.* 2009;332(1-2):145-59.

Uzuegbu UE, Onyesom I. Fructose-induced increase in ethanol metabolism and the risk of Syndrome X in man. C R *Biol.* 2009 ;332(6):534-8.

Vickers MH, Clayton ZE, Yap C, Sloboda DM. Maternal fructose intake during pregnancy and lactation alters placental growth and leads to sex-specific changes in fetal and neonatal endocrine function. *Endocrinology.* 2011 ;152(4):1378-87.

Zhang ZY, Zeng JJ, Kjaergaard M, Guan N, Raun K, Nilsson C, Wang MW. Effects of a maternal diet supplemented with chocolate and fructose beverage during gestation and lactation on rat dams and their offspring. *Clin Exp Pharmacol Physiol.* 2011 ;38(9):613-22.

In: Fructose
Editors: Brandon M. Johnston and Aaron B. Collins
ISBN: 978-1-62081-126-9

Chapter 9

MAMMALIAN TRIOKINASE AND DIHYDROXYACETONE KINASE ARE THE SAME ENZYME

David J. Timson*
School of Biological Sciences, Queen's University Belfast,
Medical Biology Centre, Belfast, UK

ABSTRACT

It is widely accepted that the ATP-dependent phosphorylation of D-glyceraldehyde in the fructokinase pathway of fructose metabolism requires the enzyme "triokinase". However, experimental data on this enzyme are remarkably scarce. The enzyme has been purified from a variety of sources and peptides derived from the pig kidney enzyme show high similarity to human dihydroxyacetone kinase – an enzyme which also has FMN cyclase activity in high manganese ion concentrations. The properties of the two enzymes are also highly similar. Therefore it is proposed that mammalian triokinase and dihydroxyacetone kinase are, in fact, the same enzyme. This has consequences for investigations of normal and aberrant fructose metabolism and for the teaching of biochemistry in medical and science courses.

INTRODUCTION: FRUCTOSE METABOLISM

Many organisms have a specialised metabolic pathway to convert the ketose monosaccharide fructose into glycolytic intermediates (Figure 1). In this pathway, fructose is first phosphorylated at position one in a reaction catalysed by fructokinase (EC 2.7.1.3) [1]. Aldolase B (EC 4.1.2.13) then catalyses the cleavage of fructose 1-phosphate into dihydroxyacetone phosphate and glyceraldehyde [1]. While dihydroxyacetone phosphate can enter glycolysis directly, glyceraldehyde needs to be phosphorylated to glyceraldehyde 3-phosphate before it can be used in this pathway. The enzyme responsible for catalysing this reaction is

* Telephone: +44(0)28 9097 5875; Fax:+44(0)28 9097 5877; Email: d.timson@qub.ac.uk

generally believed to be "triokinase" (also known as triose kinase or D-glyceraldehyde kinase; EC 2.7.1.28). Indeed this view is so well established that it is reproduced in most biochemistry textbooks (for example, see [2]). However, experimentally derived information on the structure and properties of triokinase is surprisingly sparse.

The fructokinase pathway is an important source of metabolic energy in a number of mammalian tissues, including the liver and kidney. Mutations in genes encoding fructokinase and aldolase B can result in the genetic diseases fructosuria (OMIM 229800)) and hereditary fructose intolerance (HFI; OMIM 229600) respectively [3-5]. No genetic diseases are associated with triokinase. In mammals the fructokinase pathway is only active is cells in which the concentration of glucose is high. In cells where fructose is present as the sole, or main, carbon source (eg sperm cells) then the catalysis of monosaccharide phosphorylation is carried out by hexokinase [6,7]. In some microorganisms, the genes encoding fructose metabolism are induced by the presence of fructose in the media and by the simultaneous absence of preferred carbon sources, such as glucose (for examples see [8-10]).

In recent years there has been increased interest in fructose metabolism in humans. The greater use of high fructose corn syrup (HFCS) as a sweetener in foodstuffs (especially in developed countries) has increased the dietary intake of the sugar. The consequences of this are unresolved, and controversial. While average levels of fructose intake (49 g/day in the USA [11]) do not appear to be linked to any adverse effects [12], excessive consumption may result in obesity and diabetes [13]. If fructose enters intermediate metabolism via the fructokinase pathway it bypasses one of the key control points, phosphofructokinase. High fructose intake stimulates triglyceride synthesis and accumulation and induces insulin resistance in the liver [14,15]. There is also concern about the contribution of plasma fructose to non-enzymatic glycation of proteins – especially as this sugar reacts more rapidly than the more abundant glucose [16,17]. This concern is particularly great in the case of some diabetic patients where the amounts of glucose and fructose may be approximately equal due to the operation of the polyol pathway which converts excess glucose to fructose [18].

THE REPORTED PROPERTIES OF TRIOKINASE

The isolation of an enzyme with D-glyceraldehyde kinase activity from goose liver was reported in 1953 [1]. The enzyme catalysed the phosphorylation of D-glyceraldehyde, DL-glyceraldehyde and dihydroxyacetone at approximately similar rates [1]. In the following years, the enzyme was purified from a number of sources and characterised. The pig kidney enzyme was reported to have a molecular mass of approximately 66 kDa and to form homodimers [19]. The rat liver enzyme catalyses the phosphorylation of D-glyceraldehyde and dihydroxyacetone. Its preferred substrate is ATP, but ITP and GTP can also support phosphorylation [20]. The pig liver enzyme can use ATP, CTP, GTP or UTP as a phosphate donor [19]. Both the rat and pig triokinases require magnesium ions to be present at the same concentration as the nucleotide triphosphate [19,20]. Calcium and iron (II) ions can partially substitute for magnesium, but millimolar concentrations of cobalt (II), manganese (II), nickel, copper (II) and zinc ions cannot [19].

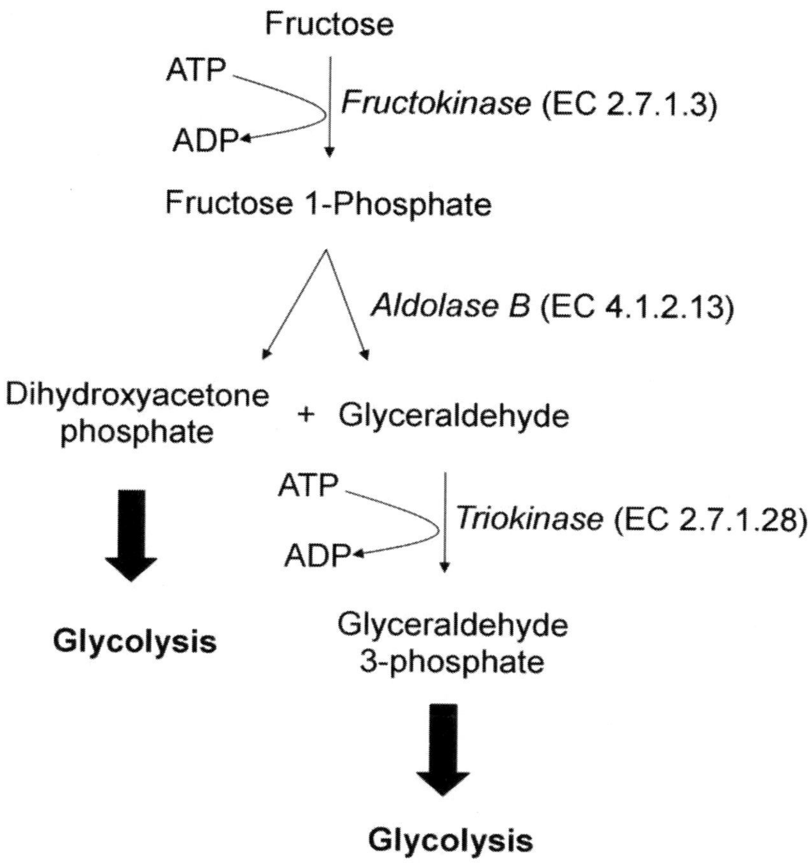

Figure 1. The fructokinase pathway of fructose metabolism. The substrates are shown in normal type and the enzymes in italics.

DIHYDROXYACETONE KINASE

The existence of an enzyme capable of catalysing the phosphorylation of another three carbon sugar, dihydroxyacetone has been reported. Dihydroxyacetone kinase (glycerone kinase; EC 2.7.1.29) activity has been isolated from a wide variety of organisms from bacteria to humans. The precise physiological role of this activity in humans, if any, is not known although it has been reported that red blood cells can metabolise dihydroxyacetone [21]. One group of bacterial dihydroxyacetone kinases are heterotetrameric; in *Escherichia coli* the complex is comprised of DhaK, DhaL and two copies of DhaM. DhaM is phosphorylated by the bacterial phosphotransferase system (PTS) with the ultimate phosphate donor being phospho*enol*pyruvate. These phosphate groups are then transferred to dihydroxyacetone in the kinase reaction [22,23]. Some other bacteria, along with plants, fungi and animals have dihydroxyacetone kinases which use ATP as a phosphate donor. Both types of enzyme have a catalytic mechanism involving a covalent enzyme-substrate complex mediated by a histidine residue in the active site [24,25]. Some microbial dihydroxyacetone kinases have also been reported to catalyse the phosphorylation of D-glyceraldehyde [24,26].

Table 1. The amino acid composition (by percentage) of pig kidney triokinase and human dihydroxyacetone kinase

Amino acid	Pig triokinase[b]	Human dihydroxyacetone kinase[c]
Ala	15.5	16.0
Arg	4.8	4.5
Asx[a]	7.3	6.1
Cys	1.2	1.0
Glx[a]	8.4	8.4
Gly	11.2	10.6
His	1.8	1.6
Ile	3.2	3.8
Leu	12.5	12.7
Lys	5.6	4.9
Met	1.3	3.0
Phe	1.5	1.4
Pro	4.3	4.2
Ser	6.7	7.5
Thr	4.9	5.0
Trp	0.7	0.9
Tyr	0.9	0.7
Val	8.4	7.8

[a] Asx represents Asn and Asp; Glx represents Gln and Glu.
[b] Experimentally determined and taken from [19].
[c] Determined from the amino acid Reference Sequence NP_056348.2 and calculated using the ProtParam program in ExPASy (http://expasy.org/cgi-bin/protparam) [32].

```
Peptide 1   LIDEG--GAAWPNVVA
            |||      |||||| |
NP_056348.2 LIDAETTAAAWPNVAA

Peptide 2       MATADEIV-HMLNHMTD
                ||||||||  ||.|||.
NP_056348.2     MATADEIVKLMLDHMTN

Peptide 3       MVRVLERVVTTLLGLEENLDAL
                |  |||||  |||||||| |.||
NP_056348.2     MALVLERVCSTLLGLEEHLNAL
```

Figure 2. Sequence alignments of the peptides obtained from pig triokinase [19].

The human enzyme is predicted to be a 575 amino acid protein of molecular mass 59 kDa (NCBI Reference Sequence NP_056348.2). This enzyme has been shown to have both dihydroxyacetone kinase and FMN cyclase (FAD-AMP lyase; EC 4.7.1.15) activity [27]. This is also the case with the enzyme from *Citrobacter freundii* where switching between the two activities appears to be regulated by the manganese (II) ion concentration. At low concentrations, kinase activity dominates; at ion concentrations above 5 mM kinase activity is almost zero, whereas FMN cyclase activity is present [28]. It has been suggested that similar, manganese ion-regulated switching may occur in other dihydroxyacetone kinases, including the human enzyme [28].

"TRIOKINASE" IS THE SAME ENZYME AS DIHYDROXYACETONE KINASE

Mammalain triokinases and dihydroxyacetone kinases share many features in common. Both have a monomeric molecular mass around 60 kDa and both probably exist *in vivo* as dimers [19,25,27]. The kinase activity of both enzymes is essentially zero in the presence of millimolar concentrations of manganese ions [19,28].

The best characterised triokinase is the one from pig kidney [19]. The amino acid composition of this enzyme is highly similar to that of the human dihydroxyacetone kinase (Table 1). Furthermore, three peptides were isolated from this sequence [19]. These sequences were tested for similarity to human protein reference sequences and, in all three cases, the most similar protein was dihydroxyacetone kinase (NP_056348.2, Figure 2). Although there is an annotated entry in the NCBI database for a human gene encoding dihydroxyacetone kinase (NM_015533.3), no such entry exists for triokinase. This combination of sequence data and enzymological evidence strongly suggests that the two enzymes are, in fact, the same molecule. Thus, the human enzyme known as dihydroxyacetone kinase is hypothesised to be capable of catalysing at least three reactions: the phosphorylation of dihydroxyacetone, the phosphorylation of D-glyceraldehyde and the cyclisation of FMN.

The peptides were aligned to human Reference Sequences using BLAST [29] as implemented on the NCBI server (www.ncbi.nlm.nih.gov/BLAST/). In each case the best match was with dihydroxyacetone kinase and these alignments are shown with ¦ representing an identical amino acid and . representing a similar one. The peptides are numbered according to the paper in which they were described [19]. Peptide 1 aligns to residues 326-341 of human dihydroxyacetone kinase. Peptide 2 aligns to residues 231-247 and peptide 3 to residues 374-395.

In work on fungal enzymes, triokinase and dihydroxyacetone kinase are often assumed to be identical – see, for example [30]. That the two mammalian enzymes are identical has been hinted at previously. The phosphorylation of dihydroxyacetone in human red blood cells was attributed to the activity of triokinase [21]. In a similar manner, the two enzymes were assumed to be identical in a study of fructose metabolism in the Purkinje fibres [31]. Furthermore, several enzyme kinetic studies suggest that dihydroxyacetone is at least as good a substrate for triokinase as D-glyceraldehyde [1,19,20]. Nevertheless, the assumption that the triokinase of the fructokinase pathway is a separate enzyme remains widespread.

The hypothesis is testable. The most elegant test would be to knock out the gene for dihydroxyacetone kinase in a mammalian model organism and test for the animal's ability to metabolise fructose to glyceraldehyde 3-phosphate in the liver (or other tissues with high glucose concentrations). However, this experiment would present some problems. The lack of FMN-cyclase activity may have significant effects and the experiment would be expensive and time-consuming to carry out. Alternatively, extracts from mammalian cells could be prepared and dihydroxyacetone kinase selectively removed by immunoprecipitation. The resulting extract should have a reduced ability to convert fructose to glyceraldehyde 3-phosphate in the presence of glucose (to ensure that hexokinase is unable to catalyse the direct phosphorylation of fructose), compared to control extracts.

Conclusion

The available evidence suggests that there are not separate enzymes in mammals with triokinase and dihydroxyacetone kinase activity. The phosphorylation of D-glyceraldehyde in fructose metabolism is carried out by dihydroxyacetone kinase – an enzyme which can also catalyse the cyclisation of FMN. Given that both glyceraldehyde and dihydroxyacetone are both trioses, the name triokinase (or triose kinase) would be appropriate as a trivial name. The exact details of how the enzyme is regulated in order to perform its three functions remain to be discovered.

References

[1] Hers, H.G. & Kusaka, T. (1953). Le metabolisme du fructose-1-phosphate dans le foie *Biochim Biophys Acta. 11,* 427-437.

[2] Berg, J.M., Tymoczko, J.L. and Stryer, L. (2011) *Biochemistry.* W.H. Freeman Palgrave Macmillan, New York, USA.

[3] Bonthron, D.T., Brady, N., Donaldson, I.A. & Steinmann, B. (1994). Molecular basis of essential fructosuria: molecular cloning and mutational analysis of human ketohexokinase (fructokinase). *Hum Mol Genet. 3,* 1627-1631.

[4] Cross, N.C., Tolan, D.R. & Cox, T.M. (1988). Catalytic deficiency of human aldolase B in hereditary fructose intolerance caused by a common missense mutation. *Cell. 53,* 881-885.

[5] Bouteldja, N. & Timson, D.J. (2010). The biochemical basis of hereditary fructose intolerance. *J Inherit Metab Dis. 33,* 105-112.

[6] Meyerhof, O. & Wilson, J.R. (1948). Studies on glycolysis of brain preparations; affinity of hexokinase for glucose and fructose. *Arch Biochem. 19,* 502-508.

[7] Jones, A. R. & Connor, D.E. (2000). Fructose metabolism by mature boar spermatozoa. *Reprod Fertil Dev. 12,* 355-359.

[8] Caescu, C.I., Vidal, O., Krzewinski, F., Artenie, V. & Bouquelet, S. (2004). *Bifidobacterium longum* requires a fructokinase (Frk; ATP:D-fructose 6-phosphotransferase, EC 2.7.1.4) for fructose catabolism. *J Bacteriol. 186,* 6515-6525.

[9] Zembrzuski, B., Chilco, P., Liu, X.L., Liu, J., Conway, T. & Scopes, R. (1992). Cloning, sequencing, and expression of the *Zymomonas mobilis* fructokinase gene and structural comparison of the enzyme with other hexose kinases. *J Bacteriol. 174,* 3455-3460.

[10] Allenza, P., Lee, Y.N. & Lessie, T.G. (1982). Enzymes related to fructose utilization in *Pseudomonas cepacia. J Bacteriol. 150,* 1348-1356.

[11] Marriott, B.P., Cole, N. & Lee, E. (2009). National estimates of dietary fructose intake increased from 1977 to 2004 in the United States. *J Nutr. 139,* 1228S-1235S.

[12] Dolan, L.C., Potter, S.M. & Burdock, G.A. (2010). Evidence-based review on the effect of normal dietary consumption of fructose on blood lipids and body weight of overweight and obese individuals. *Crit Rev Food Sci Nutr. 50,* 889-918.

[13] Tappy, L. & Le, K.A. (2010). Metabolic effects of fructose and the worldwide increase in obesity. *Physiol Rev. 90,* 23-46.

[14] Le, K.A. & Tappy, L. (2006). Metabolic effects of fructose. *Curr Opin Clin Nutr Metab Care. 9,* 469-475.

[15] Schaefer, E.J., Gleason, J.A. & Dansinger, M.L. (2009). Dietary fructose and glucose differentially affect lipid and glucose homeostasis. *J Nutr. 139,* 1257S-1262S.

[16] Suarez, G., Rajaram, R., Oronsky, A.L. & Gawinowicz, M.A. (1989). Nonenzymatic glycation of bovine serum albumin by fructose (fructation). Comparison with the Maillard reaction initiated by glucose. *J Biol Chem. 264,* 3674-3679.

[17] Dills, W.L.,Jr (1993). Protein fructosylation: fructose and the Maillard reaction. *Am J Clin Nutr. 58,* 779S-787S.

[18] Schalkwijk, C.G., Stehouwer, C.D. & van Hinsbergh, V.W. (2004). Fructose-mediated non-enzymatic glycation: sweet coupling or bad modification. *Diabetes Metab Res Rev. 20,* 369-382.

[19] Miwa, I., Kito, Y. & Okuda, J. (1994). Purification and characterization of triokinase from porcine kidney. *Prep Biochem. 24,* 203-223.

[20] Frandsen, E.K. & Grunnet, N. (1971). Kinetic properties of triokinase from rat liver. *Eur J Biochem. 23,* 588-592.

[21] Beutler, E. & Guinto, E. (1973). Dihydroxyacetone metabolism by human erythrocytes: demonstration of triokinase activity and its characterization. *Blood. 41,* 559-568.

[22] Gutknecht, R., Beutler, R., Garcia-Alles, L.F., Baumann, U. & Erni, B. (2001). The dihydroxyacetone kinase of *Escherichia coli* utilizes a phosphoprotein instead of ATP as phosphoryl donor. *EMBO J. 20,* 2480-2486.

[23] Erni, B., Siebold, C., Christen, S., Srinivas, A., Oberholzer, A. & Baumann, U. (2006). Small substrate, big surprise: fold, function and phylogeny of dihydroxyacetone kinases. *Cell Mol Life Sci. 63,* 890-900.

[24] Garcia-Alles, L.F., Siebold, C., Nyffeler, T.L., Flukiger-Bruhwiler, K., Schneider, P., Burgi, H. B., Baumann, U. & Erni, B. (2004). Phospho*enol*pyruvate- and ATP-dependent dihydroxyacetone kinases: covalent substrate-binding and kinetic mechanism. *Biochemistry. 43,* 13037-13045.

[25] Siebold, C., Arnold, I., Garcia-Alles, L. F., Baumann, U. & Erni, B. (2003). Crystal structure of the *Citrobacter freundii* dihydroxyacetone kinase reveals an eight-stranded alpha-helical barrel ATP-binding domain. *J Biol Chem. 278,* 48236-48244.

[26] Kato, N., Yoshikawa, H., Tanaka, K., Shimao, M. & Sakazawa, C. (1988). Dihydroxyacetone kinase from a methylotrophic yeast, *Hansenula polymorpha* CBS 4732. *Arch Microbiol. 150,* 155-159.

[27] Cabezas, A., Costas, M. J., Pinto, R. M., Couto, A. & Cameselle, J. C. (2005). Identification of human and rat FAD-AMP lyase (cyclic FMN forming) as ATP-dependent dihydroxyacetone kinases. *Biochem Biophys Res Commun. 338,* 1682-1689.

[28] Sanchez-Moreno, I., Iturrate, L., Martin-Hoyos, R., Jimeno, M. L., Mena, M., Bastida, A. & Garcia-Junceda, E. (2009). From kinase to cyclase: an unusual example of catalytic promiscuity modulated by metal switching. *ChemBioChem. 10,* 225-229.

[29] Altschul, S.F., Gish, W., Miller, W., Myers, E.W. & Lipman, D. J. (1990). Basic local alignment search tool. *J Mol Biol. 215,* 403-410.

[30] Bystrykh, L.V., de Koning, W. & Harder, W. (1990). Dihydroxyacetone synthase from *Candida boidinii* KD1. *Methods Enzymol. 188,* 435-445.

[31] Funari, V.A., Herrera, V.L., Freeman, D. & Tolan, D.R. (2005). Genes required for fructose metabolism are expressed in Purkinje cells in the cerebellum. *Brain Res Mol Brain Res. 142,* 115-122.

[32] Gasteiger, E., Hoogland, C., Gattiker, A., Duvaud, S., Wilkins, M.R., Appel, R.D. & Bairoch, A. (2005) Protein identification and analysis tools on the ExPASy server. In Walker, J.M. (ed.), *The Proteomics Protocols Handbook.* Humana Press, New York, USA, pp. 571-607.

INDEX

A

acetaldehyde, 118, 121, 122, 123, 125, 126, 127, 129
acetylcholine, 143
acid, 3, 5, 7, 8, 9, 18, 19, 30, 33, 34, 35, 43, 44, 50, 51, 54, 57, 58, 69, 89, 92, 96, 98, 107, 108, 119, 120, 122, 126, 127, 136, 143, 147, 150, 156
acylation, 57, 71, 74, 108
additives, x, 145
adenine, 127
adenosine, 51, 113, 134
ADH, 118, 119, 124, 125
adipocyte, 8, 13, 18, 24, 25, 26, 30, 32, 33, 57, 71, 74, 107
adiponectin, x, 5, 12, 13, 16, 17, 24, 25, 26, 33, 35, 49, 57, 71, 74, 143, 145, 150, 152
adipose, vii, ix, 1, 2, 3, 13, 18, 31, 32, 33, 35, 44, 46, 48, 49, 52, 65, 77, 82, 92, 93, 100, 107, 114, 131, 134, 135, 136, 140, 142
adiposity, 2, 29, 30, 31, 46, 49, 52, 57, 65, 66, 72, 75, 134
adolescents, 62, 63, 72
ADP, 50
adulthood, 3, 23, 25, 28, 30, 31, 86
adults, viii, 37, 38, 40, 41, 46, 48, 59, 62, 63, 67, 91, 104, 113, 141, 148
adverse effects, viii, 43, 47, 51, 52, 53, 61, 62, 105, 109, 154
aging process, ix, 101, 102, 108
alanine, 123
alcoholic cardiomyopathy, 122, 123, 130
alcoholism, 117, 120, 127, 128, 129
aldolase, viii, 38, 43, 154, 158
amblyopia, 121
American Heart Association, 33, 59, 112, 114
amines, 95
amino acid, 78, 95, 108, 112, 119, 156, 157
amniotic fluid, 44, 46
amylase, 122, 129
angiotensin II, 97, 149
anthropologists, 117
antibody, 6, 8, 85
antidepressants, 90, 99
antioxidant, 19, 26, 27, 28, 34, 90, 99, 112
anxiety, 90, 99, 143
apoptosis, 35, 149
appetite, ix, 2, 3, 16, 25, 28, 29, 32, 66, 74, 75, 76, 131, 138, 140, 142
asthma, 107
ataxia, 121
atherosclerosis, ix, 68, 101, 108
ATP, viii, x, 38, 42, 45, 51, 106, 107, 113, 123, 125, 153, 154, 155, 158, 159, 160

B

bacteria, x, 109, 145, 146, 155
beer, ix, 117, 122
benzodiazepine, 123
beverages, viii, ix, 29, 37, 38, 39, 40, 48, 49, 50, 52, 54, 56, 57, 59, 61, 62, 64, 66, 68, 70, 72, 73, 81, 82, 92, 99, 101, 102, 104, 105, 106, 110, 111, 117, 148
bicarbonate, 9
bingeing, 143
bioavailability, 52, 125
biochemistry, x, 153, 154
biomarkers, 17, 25, 33, 34, 94, 121
biosynthesis, 27
blood, ix, 4, 8, 13, 34, 42, 43, 44, 45, 46, 47, 49, 51, 52, 53, 55, 56, 58, 59, 63, 64, 67, 77, 78, 87, 89, 92, 93, 95, 96, 97, 99, 102, 103, 106, 107, 108, 110, 112, 113, 118, 119, 121, 123, 124, 125, 126, 128, 129, 131, 146, 148, 159
BMI, 62, 63, 65, 69
body composition, 132, 140, 148

body fat, 46, 49, 142
body weight, vii, x, 1, 2, 3, 30, 32, 46, 49, 50, 56, 63, 66, 71, 72, 82, 91, 99, 103, 105, 118, 124, 129, 131, 134, 140, 142, 146, 148, 149, 159
bowel, ix, 66, 101, 102, 109, 115
brain, vii, ix, 30, 34, 46, 71, 81, 83, 84, 86, 87, 89, 90, 91, 94, 95, 97, 98, 99, 118, 121, 129, 136, 142, 143, 148, 158
breast milk, 46

C

calcium, 122, 147
caloric intake, 40, 132, 133, 140, 141
calorie, 10, 12, 17, 147
cancer, 32, 107
carbohydrate(s), vii, 2, 3, 23, 24, 26, 27, 30, 31, 32, 35, 38, 39, 46, 47, 48, 50, 54, 55, 56, 72, 92, 93, 99, 103, 108, 111, 112, 113, 114, 120, 129, 145, 146, 150, 152
carbon, 39, 43, 46, 103, 119, 154, 155
carboxyl, 68, 147
carcinogenicity, 147
cardiac output, 51, 67, 122
cardiomyopathy, 122, 123, 127
cardiovascular disease, viii, ix, 2, 29, 37, 38, 48, 52, 58, 59, 60, 67, 70, 77, 81, 83, 102, 107, 108, 110, 112, 114, 129, 142, 150
cardiovascular risk, 57, 67, 100, 129
catecholamines, 89, 108
CBS, 160
C-C, 58
cDNA, 139
cecum, 146
cell culture, 51
central nervous system (CNS), ix, 29, 49, 63, 65, 71, 81, 83, 94, 127, 136, 137
central obesity, 52
cerebellum, 95, 160
cerebral cortex, 84, 90
cerebrospinal fluid, 118
chemical, viii, 7, 37, 39, 102, 122, 146
chemiluminescence, 6
children, 40, 46, 49, 57, 62, 63, 71, 82, 91, 105, 111, 112, 113, 115
cholesterol, x, 38, 43, 48, 56, 68, 77, 89, 92, 96, 97, 106, 107, 112, 120, 122, 145, 147, 148, 149
chromosome, 108
chronic diseases, vii, 2, 28, 57
circulation, 46, 51, 66, 107, 108, 119
cirrhosis, 68, 90, 128
clinical trials, 48, 68
cloning, 73, 158
clustering, 107
CO2, 5, 9, 42
cobalt, 122, 154
cocaine, 2
cognition, 90, 121
cognitive impairment, 90, 94, 96, 97, 98, 99
cognitive skills, 89
colic, 115
complex carbohydrates, 39
congestive heart failure, 122, 130
constipation, x, 145, 146, 147
consumers, 40, 41, 82, 86
consumption, vii, viii, ix, 2, 23, 24, 34, 37, 38, 40, 43, 48, 49, 51, 52, 53, 56, 59, 61, 62, 63, 64, 66, 67, 68, 69, 70, 71, 72, 79, 81, 82, 83, 84, 86, 89, 90, 91, 94, 98, 99, 100, 101, 103, 105, 106, 107, 108, 109, 110, 111, 112, 113, 115, 117, 121, 127, 129, 131, 132, 136, 140, 146, 147, 149, 151, 152, 154, 159
Continuing Survey of Food Intakes by Individuals, 142
contraceptives, 114
control group, 6, 9, 105, 132, 135, 141
controversial, 51, 119, 154
copper, 31, 154
coronary artery disease, 49, 67, 68, 103
corpus callosum, 121
corticotropin, 2, 32
covalent bond, 39
creatine, 123
CRP, 5, 12
crystalline, ix, 62, 81, 82
CSF, 118
CVD, 107
cytoplasm, 46

D

declarative memory, 84
deficiency, 65, 73, 149, 158
degradation, 77, 97, 112, 125, 143
delirium tremens, 121
dementia, 94, 150, 152
Department of Agriculture, 40, 91
deposition, 46, 49, 52, 53, 55, 62, 69, 79, 132, 140
depression, 62, 83
deprivation, 143
detoxification, 126
developed countries, 154
developing countries, 117
diabetes, viii, ix, 29, 33, 34, 35, 37, 38, 46, 48, 49, 50, 51, 52, 53, 58, 60, 62, 66, 70, 71, 81, 82, 84,

89, 91, 93, 94, 101, 102, 104, 107, 108, 110, 111, 122, 142, 151, 154
diabetic nephropathy, 115
diabetic patients, 26, 34, 104, 146, 154
diacylglycerol, 53, 107
diarrhea, ix, 41, 91, 101, 102, 109
diet, vii, ix, x, 1, 3, 6, 23, 24, 27, 30, 31, 32, 33, 34, 35, 38, 40, 43, 46, 48, 52, 53, 55, 56, 64, 66, 67, 69, 72, 73, 81, 82, 83, 84, 85, 86, 87, 88, 89, 90, 91, 92, 93, 94, 95, 96, 97, 98, 99, 100, 102, 105, 106, 107, 108, 109, 111, 112, 113, 114, 115, 131, 132, 133, 134, 136, 139, 140, 141, 142, 145, 146, 147, 149, 150, 151, 152
diffusion, 71, 118
digestion, ix, 117, 118
diseases, vii, 1, 28, 48, 50, 51, 53, 55, 71, 154
DNA, 68, 99, 108, 129
dopamine, 136, 141, 143
drinking water, 3, 6, 84, 89
dyslipemia, vii, 2
dyslipidemia, viii, 2, 37, 48, 52, 53, 55, 67, 69, 71, 73, 77, 78, 79, 92, 104, 106, 107, 108, 146, 148

E

eccentric left ventricular hypertrophy, x, 145, 151
Economic Research Service, 92
endocrine, vii, x, 1, 2, 3, 25, 27, 28, 31, 56, 73, 74, 93, 99, 145, 152
endogenous fructose production, viii, 38, 44, 45, 46
endothelial dysfunction, 52, 58, 106, 107, 113
energy, 2, 23, 29, 39, 40, 42, 43, 46, 47, 48, 49, 53, 56, 57, 63, 64, 65, 71, 72, 74, 76, 82, 89, 92, 103, 107, 108, 112, 125, 139, 142, 154
environment, viii, 2, 6, 31, 38, 44, 55, 64, 72, 96, 121
enzyme, x, 20, 26, 34, 42, 43, 63, 68, 69, 82, 83, 92, 103, 107, 118, 119, 134, 136, 153, 154, 155, 157, 158, 159
epidemic, vii, 1, 2, 29, 49, 53, 54, 58, 60, 62, 70, 72, 92, 99, 105, 132, 142
epinephrine, 97
epithelial cells, 51
erythrocytes, 26, 159
essential fatty acids, 46
estrogen, 90
ethanol, ix, x, 5, 117, 118, 119, 120, 121, 122, 123, 124, 125, 126, 127, 128, 129, 130, 145, 148, 152
ethnicity, 78
ethyl alcohol, 126
etiology, 68, 71
evolution, 41, 58
excretion, 118, 123
exercise, 38, 47, 56
exposure, 31, 66, 68, 97, 128, 134, 135, 142
extraction, 5, 146
extracts, 15, 158

F

FAD, 157, 160
family history, 46, 52, 55, 69, 79
fasting, 4, 5, 8, 43, 44, 46, 48, 49, 53, 64, 103, 105, 118
fasting glucose, 53
fat, viii, 2, 4, 5, 9, 13, 22, 24, 30, 32, 43, 48, 49, 52, 53, 61, 62, 63, 64, 66, 67, 68, 69, 70, 71, 73, 74, 87, 90, 91, 94, 95, 97, 99, 100, 103, 104, 105, 107, 109, 110, 114, 120, 126, 127, 129, 132, 134, 140, 142, 146, 147, 148, 149
fatty acids, 24, 35, 43, 44, 48, 87, 96, 103, 104, 106, 107, 108, 119, 120
female rat, 30, 31, 86, 90, 91, 93, 95
fermentation, ix, 117
fetus, viii, 38, 44, 46, 55
fibrinogen, 122
fibrosis, 52, 59, 69, 79, 126
flavonoids, 126
fluorescence, 109
fluoxetine, 90
fMRI, 87
food, vii, ix, x, 1, 3, 5, 10, 11, 15, 16, 17, 23, 24, 29, 30, 31, 44, 49, 50, 54, 62, 63, 64, 65, 66, 70, 71, 74, 89, 117, 131, 133, 134, 136, 140, 143, 145, 146, 147, 151
food intake, vii, ix, 1, 4, 5, 10, 11, 15, 16, 17, 23, 24, 29, 30, 31, 49, 50, 63, 65, 66, 71, 74, 89, 131, 134, 136, 140
food products, x, 145, 147
formation, ix, 44, 50, 98, 101, 109, 118, 122, 127, 149
fructose-rich diet (FRD), vii, 1, 3
fruits, viii, ix, 3, 38, 39, 44, 61, 62, 70, 81, 82, 101, 102, 146

G

gallstones, 107
gastrointestinal tract, x, 74, 82, 118, 145, 146
gender differences, 48, 124
gene expression, 9, 16, 24, 25, 34, 42, 68, 75, 78, 79, 94, 136, 143, 148
genes, ix, 7, 15, 50, 54, 68, 79, 104, 131, 136, 138, 139, 140, 141, 154
genetic defect, 111
genetic predisposition, 62
gestation, x, 2, 24, 30, 44, 46, 145, 150, 152

gland, 66
glucagon, 47, 122
glucocorticoid, ix, 30, 31, 131, 134, 142
gluconeogenesis, 43, 103, 120, 122, 134
glucose regulation, 95
glucose tolerance, vii, 2, 26, 27, 28, 31, 49, 52, 53, 64, 94, 105, 111, 148
GLUT4, 72, 150
glutamate, 149
glutathione, 7, 8, 26, 34, 150
glyceraldehyde, viii, x, 43, 103, 153, 154, 155, 157, 158
glycerol, viii, 38, 43, 44, 63, 103, 104, 124
glycogen, viii, 38, 43, 44, 46, 47, 103, 119, 120, 146, 150
glycolysis, 63, 82, 103, 104, 153, 158
glycosylated hemoglobin, 109
glycosylation, 27, 33, 108, 115
gout, 50, 108
growth, vii, x, 1, 28, 31, 46, 66, 74, 75, 89, 97, 143, 145, 146, 152
growth hormone, 66, 74, 75, 97, 143

H

hallucinations, 121
harmful effects, viii, x, 37, 38, 39, 46, 145
health, vii, viii, x, 2, 28, 29, 48, 61, 62, 63, 67, 70, 92, 98, 101, 103, 110, 111, 123, 132, 142, 145, 148, 151, 152
heart disease, 51, 91
heat shock protein, 122
heavy drinking, 121
hemoglobin, 108, 148
hemorrhagic stroke, 121, 127
hepatic encephalopathy, 146
hepatocellular carcinoma, 147
hepatocytes, 42, 51, 55, 63, 65, 68, 73, 82, 97, 102, 126
hepatomegaly, 90
high blood pressure, 38, 129, 146, 148
high density lipoprotein, 127
high fat, 87, 89, 90, 91, 96, 98
high manganese ion concentrations, x, 153
hippocampus, 83, 84, 87, 89, 90, 94, 98
histidine, 155
homeostasis, 2, 27, 49, 50, 54, 56, 57, 64, 71, 72, 74, 92, 108, 112, 113, 122, 148, 159
hormone(s), 25, 26, 28, 32, 49, 55, 57, 65, 71, 74, 107, 139, 107, 134, 143, 149
human health, 44, 48, 49
human immunodeficiency virus, 73
human subjects, 49, 64, 66, 67, 68
hydrogen, 26, 39, 147
hydrolysis, viii, 37, 39, 68
hydroxyl, ix, 39, 117
hyperglycaemia, 119, 120, 148
hyperglycemia, 76, 104, 107
hyperinsulinemia, ix, 3, 24, 25, 43, 54, 64, 81, 106
hyperinsulinism, 58, 76
hyperlipidemia, 52, 77, 110, 152
hyperplasia, 32
hypertension, viii, ix, x, 37, 43, 48, 49, 50, 51, 52, 53, 54, 58, 59, 60, 62, 67, 76, 81, 83, 93, 107, 110, 127, 142, 145, 148, 149, 152
hypertriglyceridemia, ix, x, 38, 43, 48, 50, 67, 68, 70, 72, 81, 90, 92, 96, 102, 103, 105, 145, 148, 152
hypertrophy, x, 32, 51, 58, 145, 149, 151
hyperuricemia, 38, 48, 50, 102
hypothalamic satiety signal, vii, 2
hypothalamus, ix, 4, 17, 32, 50, 66, 84, 97, 131, 139, 141, 143
hypothesis, 27, 46, 52, 67, 84, 87, 89, 132, 157, 158

I

immune response, x, 145, 147
immunogenetics, 61
immunoprecipitation, 158
in situ hybridization, 139
in vitro, 13, 25, 75, 92
in vivo, 66, 71, 78, 93, 109, 119, 127, 157
incidence, 62, 66, 111
incubation period, 19
individuals, vii, viii, 1, 33, 38, 50, 52, 53, 56, 61, 62, 65, 67, 68, 99, 102, 107, 119, 134, 152, 159
infants, 55, 115
infection, 149
inflammation, 24, 32, 34, 51, 52, 66, 76, 91, 94, 97, 98, 100, 106, 113, 147, 148
ingestion, vii, x, 30, 40, 41, 44, 47, 48, 49, 51, 53, 56, 58, 67, 77, 82, 91, 103, 105, 108, 109, 115, 117, 119, 123, 129, 132, 146, 151
inhibition, 3, 29, 49, 51, 58, 64, 69, 94, 97, 123
injections, 89
inositol, 44
intestine, 43, 49, 67, 102, 109, 113
intoxication, 120, 123, 124, 126, 128, 148
ions, 154, 157
irritable bowel syndrome, 109
ischemia, 86, 95, 106
isolation, 4, 154
isomerization, viii, x, 37, 145, 146

K

kidney, x, 41, 46, 50, 52, 58, 60, 66, 113, 120, 142, 145, 150, 152, 153, 154, 156, 157, 159
kinase activity, 73, 154, 157, 158
kinetics, 54, 56, 97, 157
Krebs cycle, 42

L

lactate dehydrogenase, 120
lactating mothers, vii, 1, 23, 24, 25, 28
lactation, x, 3, 10, 12, 23, 24, 25, 28, 30, 31, 145, 150, 152
lactic acid, viii, 38, 43, 51
lactose, x, 145, 146
latency, 85, 86, 88
LDL, 27, 43, 48, 55, 56, 68, 92, 107
leptin, vii, 2, 3, 4, 5, 9, 12, 13, 14, 15, 16, 17, 21, 22, 23, 24, 25, 27, 28, 29, 30, 31, 32, 33, 49, 50, 57, 65, 66, 71, 73, 74, 75, 84, 87, 88, 89, 94, 96, 103, 110, 142, 148, 151
leptin-resistance, vii, 2, 25
linoleic acid, 26
lipemia, 44, 48, 54, 104
lipid dysregulation, 77, 112
lipid metabolism, 34, 47, 54, 55, 56, 62, 64, 70, 74, 77, 89, 96, 122
lipid peroxidation, 8, 26, 33, 34, 106, 109, 129, 147
lipids, 9, 19, 27, 34, 44, 46, 48, 49, 53, 55, 56, 57, 69, 72, 90, 99, 111, 114, 118, 119, 120, 121, 126, 128, 159
lipolysis, 33, 107, 108
lipoproteins, 43, 52, 66, 76, 77, 78, 114, 120
liquid chromatography, 7, 39
liver, vii, viii, ix, 24, 27, 34, 38, 41, 42, 43, 44, 46, 47, 52, 53, 54, 59, 61, 62, 63, 64, 66, 67, 68, 69, 70, 71, 72, 73, 74, 76, 77, 78, 79, 81, 82, 88, 90, 92, 93, 95, 97, 98, 100, 101, 102, 103, 104, 105, 106, 107, 108, 110, 111, 112, 113, 118, 119, 120, 121, 122, 124, 125, 126, 128, 129, 130, 131, 134, 135, 136, 140, 142, 147, 150, 152, 154, 158, 159
liver disease, vii, viii, ix, 34, 46, 59, 61, 62, 63, 68, 70, 72, 76, 78, 79, 81, 82, 93, 95, 97, 98, 101, 102, 104, 106, 110, 111, 112, 113, 122, 129, 147, 152
low-density lipoprotein, 48, 63, 67, 68, 147, 150
LTD, 83, 89
lumen, 69, 109
lung disease, 97
lycopene, 26
lysine, 108

M

magnetic resonance, 96, 99, 106, 113
Maillard reaction, 108, 114, 159
malabsorption, 41, 54, 109, 115, 126
malnutrition, 128
mammalian cells, 154 158
manganese, x, 34, 153, 154, 157
MB, 55, 57, 70
MCP-1, 66
mellitus, 34, 102, 104, 122
membranes, 6, 102, 123
memory, ix, 81, 84, 85, 86, 87, 89, 90, 91, 94, 95, 96, 97, 98, 99
menopause, 48
meta-analysis, 48, 49
Metabolic, v, 1, 3, 10, 29, 35, 37, 41, 43, 52, 53, 54, 59, 61, 71, 73, 77, 99, 102, 107, 110, 111, 120, 129, 148, 152, 159
metabolic syndrome, vii, viii, ix, x, 1, 2, 29, 31, 33, 35, 37, 38, 43, 49, 50, 52, 53, 57, 58, 59, 60, 62, 67, 73, 75, 77, 91, 93, 100, 101, 102, 105, 106, 107, 110, 112, 113, 114, 142, 145, 148, 151
metabolism, viii, x, 23, 27, 31, 34, 37, 38, 39, 41, 42, 43, 44, 45, 46, 48, 50, 51, 52, 53, 54, 55, 62, 63, 65, 68, 70, 71, 74, 82, 89, 92, 94, 95, 96, 97, 99, 102, 103, 104, 105, 106, 110, 113, 114, 118, 119, 121, 123, 124, 125, 126, 128, 129, 140, 142, 146, 148, 153, 154, 155, 157, 158, 159, 160
metabolites, 4, 10, 12, 42, 63, 110, 147
methylene blue, 125, 126, 130
mice, 26, 33, 49, 52, 57, 59, 63, 66, 72, 76, 77, 86, 92, 95, 98, 99, 105, 111, 115
microdialysis, 141
microinjection, 95
molecular mass, 154, 157
molecular weight, ix, 117
molecules, 94, 102, 103, 108, 139
monocyte chemoattractant protein, 66
monosaccharide, viii, ix, 37, 39, 81, 82, 102, 103, 153, 154
monounsaturated fatty acids, 20
morphology, 96, 128
morphometric, 5
mortality, 114, 129
motor skills, 121
mRNA, x, 6, 9, 10, 13, 15, 16, 21, 22, 25, 27, 66, 127, 131, 134, 135, 136, 150
mRNAs, 21, 25
mutation, 67, 73, 158
mycotoxins, x, 145, 147, 152
myocardial infarction, 127
myopathy, 123, 130

N

NADH, 7, 45, 119, 120, 124, 125
National Health and Nutrition Examination Survey, 41, 63, 91, 114
necrosis, 76
nephropathy, 109
nervous system, 58, 71
neurogenesis, 84, 90, 91, 94, 98
neuroinflammation, ix, 81, 84, 90, 91, 98
neurons, 2, 25, 29, 32, 75, 84, 87, 89, 90, 141
neuropathy, 121
neuropeptides, 32
neuroprotection, 97
NH2, 73
nicotinamide, 134
nitric oxide, 51, 52, 97, 107, 147
nitrogen, 123, 127
NMR, 128
non-alcoholic fatty liver disease (NAFLD), ix, 62, 81, 83, 106
non-insulin dependent diabetes, 38
non-phosphorylated glucose, viii, 38, 45
norepinephrine, 97
Nrf2, 99
nucleotides, viii, 38, 46
nucleus, 25, 75, 136
nutrient, x, 2, 49, 103, 126, 145, 151
nutritional deficiencies, 121
nutritional status, 2, 119

O

obesity, vii, viii, ix, 1, 2, 3, 24, 25, 28, 29, 30, 31, 32, 33, 35, 37, 38, 48, 49, 50, 52, 53, 54, 58, 60, 62, 63, 64, 65, 66, 68, 70, 71, 72, 73, 76, 77, 92, 93, 99, 101, 102, 105, 107, 110, 111, 112, 132, 134, 139, 141, 142, 146, 151, 152, 154, 159
oil, 143
oleic acid, 19
omega-3, 104
optic chiasm, 4
organic compounds, ix, 117
organism, vii, 2, 38, 50, 158
organs, 66, 119, 127
overproduction, 26, 67, 68, 76, 77, 97, 112, 127
overweight, 24, 28, 32, 38, 49, 50, 52, 55, 57, 62, 63, 64, 72, 99, 104, 105, 111, 112, 159
oxidation, 26, 33, 34, 39, 47, 54, 55, 56, 66, 105, 118, 119, 120, 121, 123, 124, 125, 126, 129, 147
oxidative damage, 27, 33, 149
oxidative stress, vii, ix, 1, 2, 3, 30, 31, 34, 35, 51, 52, 53, 59, 81, 83, 84, 90, 91, 94, 96, 97, 98, 99, 128, 147
oxygen, viii, 38, 39, 55, 98, 149

P

pancreas, 35, 82, 128
pancreatitis, 122
parenchymal cell, 118
pathogenesis, ix, 27, 30, 58, 60, 67, 68, 70, 73, 77, 78, 99, 101, 102, 106, 108, 114, 115, 147
pathology, 70
pathophysiology, 52, 53, 114, 149
PCR, 5, 6, 7, 9, 22, 137, 139, 141
peptides, x, 31, 49, 50, 78, 139, 153, 156, 157
perfusion, 105
perinatal, 46
peripheral blood, 46, 147
peripheral neuropathy, 121
peroxidation, 106
peroxynitrite, 127
pH, 4, 8, 9
pharmaceutical, 146
phenol, 5
phenotype, vii, 2
phosphate, viii, 5, 8, 38, 43, 63, 92, 103, 104, 106, 122, 125, 134, 153, 154, 155, 158
phosphoenolpyruvate, 155
phospholipids, viii, x, 37, 38, 46, 145, 147
phosphorus, 106, 113, 114
phosphorylation, x, 17, 25, 27, 43, 51, 53, 64, 65, 66, 72, 78, 83, 84, 89, 94, 96, 106, 108, 122, 153, 154, 155, 157, 158
physical activity, 72, 111
physical inactivity, 64, 70
pioglitazone, 94
pituitary gland, 66
placenta, 44, 66
placental barrier, 46
plants, vii, 38, 39, 44, 146, 155
plasma levels, 8, 12, 17, 68, 97, 150
plasminogen, 5, 33, 98, 107
plasticity, ix, 29, 81, 98
platelet aggregation, 107, 122
plexus, 8
polyacrylamide, 6
polymers, 39, 47
polymorphism, 50, 111
polyunsaturated fat, 20
polyvinylidene fluoride, 6
potential benefits, 152
pregnancy, x, 3, 29, 31, 55, 145, 152

preschool, 62, 105, 112
prevention, 59, 71, 72, 146
probiotic, x, 145, 147
pro-inflammatory, 52
proliferation, x, 51, 90, 97, 145, 147
prostate gland, 44
protein kinase C, 27, 53
proteins, 5, 10, 33, 43, 69, 79, 83, 89, 99, 103, 108, 115, 122, 150, 154
PTEN, 108
public health, vii, 1, 28, 49

R

race, 132
reactions, 33, 42, 108, 118, 157
reactive oxygen, 3, 118, 147, 148, 149
receptors, x, 33, 49, 78, 94, 131, 139, 141, 148
red blood cells, 155, 157
regeneration, viii, 38
regression model, 56, 99
reinforcement, 86
relaxation, 52, 149
resistance, vii, x, 2, 25, 28, 30, 34, 46, 51, 52, 58, 64, 65, 74, 84, 89, 91, 94, 96, 106, 107, 145, 148
response, 23, 24, 25, 26, 31, 50, 51, 52, 65, 66, 68, 69, 73, 74, 89, 93, 94, 96, 97, 98, 99, 104, 107, 108, 135, 141, 142, 149
reticulum, 35, 69, 79, 98, 118, 122
retinol, 26
risk factors, 105, 107, 112
RNA, 4, 5, 9, 136
rodents, viii, ix, 37, 46, 52, 66, 75, 79, 81, 82, 87, 89, 146

S

saliva, 118, 129
Salmonella, 146
saturated fat, 34, 79, 96
saturation, 47
secretion, 3, 13, 23, 28, 33, 42, 47, 48, 49, 50, 51, 54, 55, 63, 65, 66, 68, 69, 74, 75, 76, 77, 78, 79, 92, 93, 104, 105
sedentary behavior, 49, 64
seed, x, 39, 145, 150, 152
self-esteem, 62
seminal vesicle, 44
serine, 27, 74, 84
serum, x, 12, 24, 25, 27, 28, 31, 32, 35, 51, 66, 78, 96, 103, 108, 109, 112, 122, 123, 128, 129, 145, 147, 159
serum albumin, 159
sex, x, 31, 145, 151, 152
sham, 143
sheep, 46, 55
signalling, x, 145, 150, 152
signals, 16, 24, 76
silica, 97
skeletal muscle, 3, 30, 52, 65, 72, 79, 107, 123, 150
sleep deprivation, 99
sleep disturbance, 107
small intestine, 41, 47, 50, 52, 113, 118, 146, 151
sodium, 6, 47, 51
solution, 3, 4, 5, 6, 8, 41, 47, 49, 84, 87, 125, 132, 133, 134, 135, 136, 138, 139, 140, 143
sperm, 3, 154
Sprague-Dawley rats, 3, 93, 100, 133
stability, 151
stabilization, 6
starch, viii, 31, 37, 39, 48, 71, 105, 108, 112, 140
starvation, 103, 107, 120
sterile, 4, 8, 9
stimulation, 24, 42, 51, 53, 65, 66, 122, 128
stimulus, 23
stomach, 50, 66, 74, 75, 118, 125
storage, 63, 86, 90, 103, 148
stress, 34, 35, 65, 69, 70, 73, 77, 79, 90, 91, 98, 99, 112
stress response, 77, 112
striatum, 136, 143
substrate, 27, 32, 53, 56, 65, 66, 83, 106, 108, 113, 150, 154, 155, 157, 159
substrates, 55, 63, 104, 155
sucrose, vii, viii, ix, 2, 24, 27, 33, 34, 37, 38, 39, 40, 41, 44, 46, 48, 49, 53, 54, 55, 56, 58, 71, 76, 81, 82, 91, 93, 102, 104, 105, 106, 107, 108, 109, 110, 111, 112, 113, 123, 131, 132, 133, 134, 136, 140, 141, 142, 143, 146, 148, 151, 152
supplementation, x, 49, 145, 152
suppression, 49, 57, 74, 110, 141, 142, 147
sweeteners, viii, x, 37, 40, 41, 53, 110, 132, 145, 146, 151
sympathetic nervous system, 51, 149
synaptic plasticity, 83, 98
syndrome, 29, 50, 51, 52, 56, 74, 77, 94, 102, 106, 107, 108, 110, 121, 129, 148
synovial fluid, 118
synthesis, vii, viii, 38, 42, 43, 44, 46, 50, 58, 63, 92, 103, 105, 120, 136, 143, 147, 154
systolic blood pressure, 50

T

tachycardia, 58
therapy, 73, 97, 123, 126

threonine, 74, 84
thyroid, 143
thyrotropin, 2, 143
tissue, 2, 3, 9, 25, 27, 28, 33, 44, 55, 107, 118, 123, 129, 134, 136, 142
TNF, x, 12, 24, 52, 66, 108, 131, 139, 143, 147
total cholesterol, 5, 10, 25, 48
toxic effect, 50, 51, 122, 128, 152
toxicity, 35, 121
transcription, 5, 6, 53, 60, 65, 68, 78, 84, 94
transducer, 5, 6, 65, 84
trial, 52, 69, 105, 112, 126, 147
tricarboxylic acid, 43
tricarboxylic acid cycle, 43
triggers, vii, 2, 68
triglycerides, viii, ix, 17, 19, 24, 25, 38, 44, 48, 49, 53, 56, 57, 67, 74, 78, 82, 89, 92, 110, 131, 132, 136, 140, 142, 148, 150
tumor, 5, 52, 59, 76, 84, 90, 108, 143
tumor necrosis factor, 5, 52, 59, 76, 84, 90, 108, 143
type 2 diabetes, vii, 1, 2, 55, 56, 57, 59, 63, 68, 69, 70, 72, 79, 94, 99, 100, 102, 104, 105, 107, 111, 114, 143, 146, 148
tyrosine, 27, 53, 64, 65, 66, 72, 77, 83, 89, 94, 107, 113, 143

U

umbilical cord, 46, 55
unhealthy diets, vii, 1, 2
uric acid, 50, 51, 57, 58, 75, 93, 107, 108, 113, 114, 128, 148, 149
urine, 32, 118
USDA, 40, 54
uterus, 55

V

vasculature, 121
vasoconstriction, 51
vasodilation, 51
vasodilator, 51
vegetables, viii, ix, 3, 37, 38, 41, 81, 82, 101, 103
very low density lipoprotein, 77, 78, 97, 103, 112
visceral adiposity, ix, 57, 64, 72, 81, 104, 111
vitamin E, 99
vitamins, 70, 126
VLDL, 27, 43, 44, 46, 48, 63, 66, 67, 68, 69, 76, 77, 78, 103, 104

W

water, ix, 3, 4, 6, 39, 49, 64, 67, 69, 84, 85, 86, 90, 94, 95, 109, 118, 119, 124, 131, 132, 133, 134, 136
wealth, 83
weight gain, 2, 29, 56, 64, 70, 74, 94, 110, 111, 132, 140
weight loss, 50, 132
western blot, 15, 83
white blood cells, 34
World Health Organization (WHO), 1, 111, 117, 130
worldwide, vii, viii, 1, 2, 28, 37, 49, 52, 53, 59, 71, 152, 159

Z

zinc, 32, 154